GETTING THE BEST FOR YOUR CHILD
WITH AUTISM

Getting the Best for Your Child with Autism

AN EXPERT'S GUIDE TO TREATMENT

BRYNA SIEGEL, PhD

THE GUILFORD PRESS
New York   London

To David

© 2008 The Guilford Press
A Division of Guilford Publications, Inc.
72 Spring Street, New York, NY 10012
www.guilford.com

Printed in the United States of America

This book is printed on acid-free paper.

Last digit is print number: 9   8   7   6   5   4   3   2   1

Library of Congress Cataloging-in-Publication Data
Siegel, Bryna.
   Getting the best for your child with autism: an expert's guide to treatment / by Bryna Siegel.
      p. cm.
   Includes bibliographical references and index.
   ISBN-13: 978-1-59385-317-4 (pbk.: alk. paper)
   ISBN-10: 1-59385-317-3 (pbk.: alk. paper)
   ISBN-13: 978-1-59385-601-4 (hardcover: alk. paper)
   ISBN-10: 1-59385-601-6 (hardcover: alk. paper)
   1. Autism in children—Treatment—Popular works.   I. Title.
   RJ506.A9S528 2008
   649'.154—dc22

                                                                    2007021759

Contents

Acknowledgments

The truths about autism that are told here are amalgamated from the observations of many people, as well as from the expected sources of empirical data. Research data tells only some of the true story about autism, and the state of the art for helping children with autism is still something that can be best practiced after seeing how "the data" play out in the experiences of those who "live," and "do" autism every day. Those that "live" and "do" autism are the ones I want to thank here:

A Thank-You to Parents I Know

The main impetus to write this book was to help try to make the lives of parents of children with autistic spectrum disorders easier, better, and more fulfilling. I gratefully acknowledge the parents of all the children I have had the pleasure to come to know. Not only do I have the opportunity for in-depth meetings with parents in my clinic, I also have the privilege of meeting parents throughout the country as I travel and lecture. Parents are always presenting me with "diamonds in the rough": insights about their children that sparkle with life when aligned with data from one kind of study or another, making that truth come alive, and allowing it to become a facet of a greater understanding I can use to help others by sharing it. I thank each of you.

A Thank-You to Teachers I Know

Broadly defined, everyone who thinks of how to make something more meaningful to a child is that child's teacher. In writing this book,

I've tried to take the perspective of special education teachers, general education teachers, and specialists such as speech and language pathologists and occupational therapists. I've learned so much from how your training and experiences, different from my own, can be invaluable in shaping my own thinking. A very special *mahalo* to a particularly masterful group of teachers: the Yo-Yo Sisterhood of Oahu—you know who you are!

A Thank-You to My Students and Colleagues

Day-to-day, much of my work on autism is done in the context of my clinic, the Autism Clinic at the Children's Center at Langley Porter, which is part of the University of California, San Francisco. At the heart of this clinic is its clinical coordinator, Monica Arroyo, and associate director, Dr. Eva Ihle, who succeed my close professional colleague of many years, Dr. Glen Elliott. In addition, the Autism Clinic consists of an ever-changing crew of volunteers who are (soon-to-be) teachers and therapists, as well as child psychiatrists and child neurology trainees. These trainees of the last few years are too numerous to list here, but my thanks go to them all, especially Drs. Miriam King and Ariella Popple Heidecker, Jannicke Stav, Lisa Schmidt, Cassandra Chaves, and Katie Pedgrift. In addition to the Autism Clinic staff, I also thank my professional colleagues who sustain me with always evolving discussions, including Dr. Elysa Marco here at UCSF Pediatric Neurology, Drs. Adriana Schuler and Pamela Wolfberg from San Francisco State University, and Dr. Felice Parisi, who was critical in initiating the JumpStart Learning-to-Learn program. Dr. Michelle Ficcaglia, director of JumpStart Learning-to-Learn, has been critical in implementing my vision for directly helping parents of newly diagnosed children. I have also learned immensely from key JumpStart founding staff—Gerry Fabella (on communication development), Andrew Shahan (on play and social interaction), and Erin Griswold (on motivation and direct teaching), all of whom are stellar, gifted therapists.

Finally, thanks to Kitty Moore at The Guilford Press, who approached me several years ago to write this book. I thank her and the superb editor Chris Benton for keeping me moving through this process.

Introduction

This is a book for parents who already know a thing or two about autism. You probably already realize that as the parent of a child who has or may have an autism spectrum disorder (autism, Asperger syndrome, or pervasive developmental disorder not otherwise specified [PDDNOS]), you'll need to learn some extra-ordinary skills to deal with this situation you now find yourself in. You're going to need new expertise on how your child sees the world and how he can learn. You're going to have to analyze all kinds of therapy and special education services available out there and figure out which ones might be what your child needs most. You're going to need a new kind of understanding about parenting—not just to deal with any problem behaviors, but importantly, to proactively "wrap around" all your child's treatments to make what's happening in them meaningful and motivating in your child's everyday life so every moment becomes a chance for your son or daughter to get better.

In this book, I'll help you understand your child's relative strengths and weaknesses so you'll understand how stronger abilities can be used to bring up the weaker areas (Chapter 6). We'll talk about many kinds of treatments and treatment strategies for autism (Chapters 7 and 8). Then, equipped with this knowledge of your child's strengths and weaknesses, you can hook up with the treatments and treating professionals who can help *your* child best. To make sure you can get treatment going smoothly, we'll talk about how you can recognize the "best fit" therapists, teachers, programs, and schools for your child

(Chapter 10). We'll talk about your legal rights as a parent of a child with autism—so you know what your child is entitled to and how to ensure that your child's rights are protected and honored (Chapter 9).

When you finish this book, I want you to feel you are absolutely equipped to be the best parent you can be for your child with autism. What do I mean by that? Well, this: If, instead of autism, your child had been diagnosed with diabetes, cystic fibrosis, or even severe asthma, you'd have to read, take classes, and talk to different kinds of doctors and therapists to learn what to do to get the best possible care for your child. You'd have to find the right kinds of doctors and therapists, learn to administer tests and medicines, be trained to watch for signs of a downturn, and create an environment at home where a specific diet or an allergen-free environment gave your child the best chance of living symptom-free. Parents of children with a physical condition have many more resources out there to give them the training they need. With that in mind, this book was written to prepare you to be the same sort of specialist in caring for your child with autism. Instead of becoming an expert at testing insulin levels and measuring carbohydrates, you're going to become an expert at sussing out the right therapists and teachers and at parenting your child so that you boost the work they do by motivating him to use his developing abilities.

I'll teach you the special principles that govern how children with autism learn. I'll show you how to make sure *your* child's *specific* needs are identified through the right kinds of assessment, and then how to navigate through many different systems of care, support, and resources to get what your individual child will require to grow and develop to the best of his or her potential. All children with autism spectrum disorders have slightly to very different difficulties, and therefore will have different treatment needs. You as the parent are in the strongest position to ensure that your child's program is individualized appropriately. There is all sorts of information out there about autism, and this book will provide you with some ideas for sorting the wheat from the chaff (Chapter 5).

Who Exactly Is This Book For?

This book is for you if you've either learned your child has autism or strongly suspect your child has some form of autism. It's for you if you feel you're going to need a bit more help to get things started—*or* really change what is already happening to help your child. Sure, there is always more you can learn. So, how do you appraise whether what you know now is enough to get started?

Read Part I of this book if you're still thinking about the diagnosis—whether it's right, and what sense you're supposed to make of having simply been told, "Yes, your child is autistic." Chapter 2 will tell you what a good diagnostic assessment should give you. In fact, if you aren't that far along yet, Chapter 1 is about screening for autism and will help you know whether you really have something to be concerned about—and whether you need someone with more expertise to help you decide that. If you've had a diagnosis, did it seem right? Do you feel you need or want a second opinion? Did you get all your questions answered? Do you need help gathering your thoughts and organizing those questions so you can approach an(other) assessment well informed?

Maybe you're farther along. If you're done with diagnosis and assessment, you might start with Part II of this book: Do you already know enough to get started with treatment? What kinds of services is your child entitled to anyway? How do you get those services? How do you know if services you have are the right ones or if they are working the way they are supposed to? How do you take the knowledge you've gathered so far and apply it to making your child's life better?

In my earlier books on autism I've tried to help parents and teachers understand who their child with autism is and how their child learns. In *The World of the Autistic Child: Understanding and Treating Autistic Spectrum Disorders*, I've written about understanding what makes for the diagnosis of autism, what getting a diagnosis involves, and how to understand treatment. In *What about Me?: Siblings of Developmentally Disabled Children*, my colleague Stu Silverstein and I talked about how autism and other disabilities affect siblings, marriages, and the whole family. In *Helping Children with Autism Learn: Treatment Approaches for Parents and Professionals*, my latest book, I wrote about how each symptom of autism can really be seen as its own type of autistic learning disability, how different treatments may address some but not other autistic learning disabilities, and how parents and teachers need programs that cover all these autistic-type learning difficulties when designing an individualized treatment plan for a child with autism.

Now, in this book, I've put it all together to help you get the best for your child with autism. I draw on all my past writings, which themselves are based on more than twenty-five years of working with children on the autism spectrum as a researcher, diagnostician, educator, and treatment program consultant. In my years in this field I've worked with autistic children, their families, and their treatment providers in many capacities. I have a rather polyglot professional identity—with an undergraduate degree in clinical psychology, a master's in early childhood education, a doctorate in child development (applied studies of children), with a doctoral minor in developmental psychology (more theoretical and empirical studies of children). On top of that, I did postdoctoral research training to hone in on methods especially applicable to bettering our understanding of autism. For almost twenty years I've been a professor in a department of psychiatry and a faculty member in a child psychiatry program. So, I speak the languages of many different professions. I feel like a bit of a cultural anthropologist in the role of a "participant observer," pretty much passing myself off as a clinical psychologist when among clinical psychologists, as an educator when I am with educators, and as a "native speaker" among child psychiatrists. This has enabled me to draw readily on all these areas of endeavor to understand children with autism and their families, and particularly to understand the special learning processes we see in children on the autism spectrum. For almost twenty years, I've been doing research and running a large diagnostic and treatment planning clinic I founded in 1989 at the University of California, San Francisco: I have seen close to 4,000 children with autism spectrum disorders.

There are many questions that I have found parents ask when they worry or find out that their child has an autism spectrum disorder. Some questions will have to do with the child himself, but others are about what this will mean to them as this child's parents—and as the individuals who existed before they became parents of a child with autism. What will autism mean for our marriage? For other children we have or may have? How will my child be seen by grandparents and our other relatives? How do I explain this to them? These topics will be addressed in Chapter 4.

Very likely, you will also have questions about the health care system, including the doctors who make diagnoses and develop treatment plans, and then the therapists who provide individualized services like speech and language therapy or occupational therapy; these questions will be addressed in Chapter 3. Following close behind your time learning from health care providers will be your time to start understanding therapies and education and the laws and entitlements you need to know about when you have a child with special needs. In this book, as you learn to travel through these different new areas of your life, I'll try to be your navigator.

Doing Everything You Can

As your child grows, develops, changes, and improves, how do you know what to expect? It's natural for parents to wish for their child to be "cured." Parents of young children with autism wish for this a lot. No one wants to take away hope. Everyone wants to encourage dreams. Your child is *your* child. You love her because she is yours. She is a part of you.

Evolution has endowed parents of any species with the most tenacious of drives for seeing to the perpetuation of that species. However, it is only the human that is endowed with a massive frontal cortex—the thinking, reasoning part of the brain. We human parents therefore seek to use this unique endowment to do all we can for our children. However, more often than not, there will be things we can't accomplish, try as we might. I'm going to help you try your best so you can do as much as possible to enable your child to fulfill his potential.

No one asks to be the parent of a child with autism. No one says to his or her husband or wife, "Well, we've got a boy and a girl; let's have one more and try for an autistic child this time. It could be *so* rewarding! There is *so* much we could learn!" Autism, and all the extra burdens of care, are thrust upon each and every person whose life it enters. Several years ago, I was on a traveling lecture panel for California Early Start (a delivery system for federally mandated services for children from birth through age three). Another panelist was the mom of a ten-year-old boy with autism. She would always begin her lecture with a story she had read in an issue of *The Advocate*, the newsletter of the Autism Society of America. The story was about a woman who had long planned a trip to France because she loved good wine and French food and had learned to speak French. One day, she finally had an opportunity to go on her long-awaited trip. When the airplane landed, though, she found she was in Holland, not France. The woman was disappointed, and although she had not planned for Holland and knew nothing about it, she realized she could learn. They didn't have vineyards, but they had charming windmills. They didn't speak French, which she had studied for such a long time, but Dutch. The mother who told this story was really a wonderful person: She said that she loved it because she found it a fitting metaphor for finding oneself the parent of a child with autism. She felt that she had learned that Holland was a place where she could be quite comfortable living. This book is about learning to live in a new place, at home with autism.

PART I

Mapping the Road to the Best Treatment

HOW TO GET
A THOROUGH DIAGNOSIS

There's no doubt: The primary purpose of any diagnosis is to lead to appropriate treatment. This is why I've devoted the first three chapters of this book to the diagnostic process. Without a thorough, expert evaluation that starts with a diagnosis and ends with an individualized treatment plan, you're stopped cold right in the entrance to the maze that winds through a confusing array of treatment and educational options available to kids with autism. Getting a diagnosis should really help in explaining why your child does many of the odd things she does and why she doesn't do the things you thought she would. An assessment, or multiple assessments, of your child will help you learn how your child sees the world. With this understanding you can help her use new skills *and* start learning the things that others her age already know.

Unfortunately, many parents of children who end up diagnosed with autism endure false starts and spend time lost in the maze when early contact with helping professionals hasn't afforded an opportunity to develop a crucial understanding about how their particular child has the best chance to overcome as many of his difficulties as he possibly can. This is why, even though many of you have already received a diagnosis of an autism spectrum disorder for your child, it can be important to retrace your steps to make sure you've had key questions answered: Does the diagnosis make sense to you considering what you know about how your child learns? Has it answered your questions about the observations that raised your concerns to begin with? Has your child changed significantly since the diagnosis was rendered, making you wonder if the same conclusion would be reached if the child were evaluated today? Did the diagnosis lay out a clear path to treatment? If you answer no to any of these questions, you'll want to read this section and consider whether to pursue further evaluation.

What makes a diagnostic assessment good (beyond being covered by your medical insurance)? What questions will you want to be sure you have answered? What can you expect to learn from a diagnostic assessment? How should you prepare for it so that you'll get all your questions answered? What should you be learning from a diagnostic assessment about your child's individual treatment needs?

Even if you're confident that you've gotten an accurate, expert diagnosis that points the way to specific treatments that will help address your child's specific symptoms, the following chapters will help you take full advantage of the diagnostic findings you've been given—like interpretations of tests, rating scales, and behavioral assessments—in all their detail, in order to craft interventions for your child's evolving needs. And, of course, if you have yet to seek an evaluation but have been concerned about your child for some time and what you've read has confirmed your worries, this section will help you start out on the right foot in getting the careful assessment your child deserves.

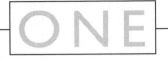

ONE

Off to a Good Start

TIMELY SCREENING WILL SET YOU
ON THE PATH TO HELP

You can get to the best treatment plan for your child with autism by a number of paths, but they all start with screening followed up by a good diagnostic visit. Autism cuts across many domains of a child's development, and available treatments tackle the disorder from all different angles. As a parent, you'll soon learn that the challenge in getting the right help for your child is that not all children are affected in each domain in exactly the same way. So if you want to make sure that a treatment plan will be designed to fit your unique child, you need to get a very complete diagnostic picture.

But when should you get started? It doesn't take a lot of reading about autism to know that kids with these disorders need a lot of help and that the earlier you get started, the better off your child is likely to be. So you may be very eager to have your child assessed—yet wonder how much a doctor can tell you about a one-year-old. Or maybe you've already taken your concerns to your pediatrician and been told to "wait and see," and you don't know if you should. Perhaps you've had your child screened and been told your child may very well have autism and now you have no idea where to go for help—or what kind of help to seek. Or the doctor said your child probably doesn't have autism but you're still quite worried that he does. Now what?

This chapter is about what to do with your earliest concerns that your child might have autism. It will tell you how to get a reliable screening—and what the key early signs of autism are. If your earliest concerns arose a long time ago, and you've already started following up on them, you may very well be more interested in the next leg of this journey—how to arrive at the best treatment plan and then put it in place. You may not need to read about screening, but I urge you to read this chapter to make sure you know what questions you will need to have answered by a diagnostic visit. A thorough, targeted diagnostic assessment is essential to arriving at a good treatment plan. A good diagnosis should not just tell you whether or not your child has autism but also help you understand your particular child's current development levels, motivators, learning strengths, and learning weaknesses. If you realize that whatever evaluations you've already had have left gaps in the information needed to address your child's weaknesses and capitalize on his strengths, you may want to seek further assessments that help you understand these things. So whether you've been down this road before or are just setting out, you can use this chapter to make sure the necessary groundwork is solid.

Screening and Referral: The First Steps

Once most parents feel certain that they have reason to be concerned about their child, they'll first consult a primary care professional—like their pediatrician or family doctor. These doctors can *screen* a child for autism as the first step in determining whether a more detailed assessment will be necessary and will send you on to someone qualified to reach a diagnosis.

What Does "Screening" Mean?

It's important to realize that a "positive" screen by a pediatrician is not the same thing as a diagnosis. A positive screen is really just a "ticket" to see a specialist. The purpose of screening for autism is to determine whether the child has enough risk factors for the disorder to justify a more intensive, extensive, expensive assessment, which should involve observation, testing, and history taking specifically for autism by someone trained to do that type of assessment. (Screening usually involves just a pencil-and-paper questionnaire and is really a "rough estimate" of what might be wrong.) Autism screening is designed to overinclude children who might have some form of autism but will need a full assessment to find out if they do have it. Obviously, it's important to be sure your child has been screened well; otherwise he might be excluded from a more thorough assessment that he needs. If you have any doubts about the screening process your child has already undergone—or wonder whether your primary care doctor can perform this screening—use the information in this chapter to start over or start right.

Autism screening is an area where there is a growing amount of research. Much of my own research work, namely, development of an early parent-reported screening test for autism—the PDDST-II (Pervasive Developmental Disorders Screening Test)—as well as other early screening tests for autism spectrum disorders like the CHAT (Checklist for Autism in Toddlers) and M-CHAT (Modified CHAT) can specifically identify unique traits that mark the earliest form of autism. The emphasis in a screener is on *unique* traits of autism and the presence of multiple concerns—as some other screeners include lots of questions that are true of children with autism but are not particularly unique to autism—and therefore a screening test can lead you into thinking your child has autism when he doesn't. Each of the screeners I mentioned is basically a short questionnaire for parents to report on key concerns about their child who might have autism. Depending on the screener used, the age of the child, the experience of the parent, and the review of the screener by a professional, the screener, used properly, can be exceedingly helpful in getting a child into the diagnostic "pipeline."

Is the Pediatrician in a Good Position to Screen Your Child?

A pediatrician or family doctor who isn't familiar with autism or doesn't use a particular screener should send you straight to an audiologist, a speech therapist, or an early interventionist—who will surely be able to do this. If the primary care doctor doesn't refer you—or you have misgivings about the results of the screening—call a speech and language pathologist, the special education intake services in your school district, or the child psychiatry program of a local university or medical center and self-refer your child. Whoever you talk to will likely take your concerns seriously, ask questions, and then explain whether and where there is a place to go next. At this point, don't worry about referral channels or insurance coverage; just try to get your child seen. You can always "reverse engineer" the paperwork after an appointment is scheduled.

One thing to know is that a large percentage of families I see in our clinic have been told, at least once, not to worry. When they do find out their child has autism, they understandably feel frustrated that the pediatrician brushed off their initial concerns. If you're in this position, you may feel angry, but know that it's not the end of the world. Not knowing about autism likely does not reflect on your pediatrician's competence in the areas of physical growth and development—so this doctor may still very well be the best choice for well-baby care.

While the American Academy of Pediatrics is placing more emphasis on all primary care doctors being able to screen for autism and related conditions, pediatric training for most doctors gives them few opportunities to learn much about developmental disorders like autism. Although you may be surprised to learn this, it has only been in the past ten years or so that screening for specific developmental or psychiatric disorders has even appeared on the pediatric training "radar." On top of this, many primary care doctors have practices that simply don't allow enough time during a well-baby check to do much in the way of addressing a parent's developmental concerns. This is why screeners for autism like the PDDST-II are designed to be filled out in a pediatric waiting room and then take only an additional five minutes of the doctor's time if it looks like the test is positive. They are specifically designed for the busy doctor without much special knowledge of autism, who may need a positive "test" to justify the cost of further special evaluation to his HMO or PPO organization.

This is also why you should educate yourself about the screening process. If you know what a screening should do and which concerns may indicate that your child has autism, you'll know whether you've gotten on the right track.

"Should I Try to Screen My Child for Autism Myself?"

Of course a little knowledge can be a dangerous thing. Many proactive parents, when they start to investigate their concerns that their child may have autism, naturally go to the Internet to search for "autism" and "screening," possibly turning up the PDDST-II or CHAT. But there are a couple of concerns here. All of us who have worked on the development of early screeners for autism can agree that getting a parent report of first concerns is where we must start. Parents see their child in more situations than any doctor or other professional, know what the child's consistent personality traits are, and can tell whether a particular worrisome form of behavior may sometimes occur—even if it doesn't occur often. However, the parents' reports must be put into context by a professional who can weight the behaviors reported in the context of other children with autism. The parent who has read about autism has not had the opportunity to meet many autistic children at different ages and so is not in a particularly good position to assess what is "typical" of autism. That means that screening for autism, just like everything else that will come after, must be a collaboration between parent and professional. For your part, you can gather the observations that have been worrying you to take to the primary care doctor. If you've already had your child screened, make sure you and the doctor covered this ground.

How Early Is Early Enough—or Too Early?

One of the first things parents worry about when they see signs that something may be wrong with their child is when to seek professional advice. If your child has already been screened, you may wonder if you had this done at the right time. Was it too early for any definitive answer to be given? Can you be sure the outcome of the screening was accurate if done too early? On the other hand, you may worry that you or your pediatrician waited too long and this denied your child the earliest possible treatment.

A well-trained clinician can pick up autism by twenty-four months of age, and some very specialized clinicians can pick it up by eighteen months of age. Before that age, a child may be missing language milestones (like communicative use of babbling)—which might be autism or might be something else, like a severe language impairment. In either case, bringing the baby to the attention of a professional should help the child get started on services he can use (like language therapy) irrespective of the diagnosis. Anybody who claims to be certain of a diagnosis of autism at fourteen months old or younger has more self-confidence than direct familiarity with the research literature. There may be interventions you want to start below one and a half years old—we'll certainly talk about that—but developmental rates and patterns are so uneven in the first couple of years that we are not always positive exactly what we are treating.

Keep in mind that recognizing autism early is not as easy as getting your child's primary care provider to administer an early screening test. A screening test is just that, *screening*, not *diagnosis*. As I said earlier, a screening test is an indication that a careful, detailed assessment must be done to determine whether the child has some form of autism and, if so, what kind of treatment plan will be the best fit. I'm repeating this because many parents I meet have gotten the false impression that their child was "diagnosed" with autism using a screening test like the PDDST-II or the CHAT, or even a screening test that is *not* specifically designed for toddlers and very young children like the CARS (Childhood Autism Rating Scale), which school psychologists sometimes use, or the GARS (Gilliam Autism Rating Scale), which is newer than the CARS but has very low specificity (that is, ability to describe symptoms uniquely associated with autism).

A large percentage of children with severe early language disorders, mental retardation, or a language problem or developmental disability plus a problem like severe anxiety or attentional problems can screen "positive" for autism on a screening test. So—don't start thinking of your child as "autistic" until your child has undergone a full diagnostic evaluation and received a definitive diagnosis from a specialist diagnostician. Depending on which screening test is used, about 75% to 90% of children who are screened positive will turn out to have some sort of autism spectrum disorder. While those are pretty good statistics for screening any sort of disorder, it also means that 10% to 25% of children for whom the screener raised concerns about autism were not really autistic at all.

Early Signs Most Unique to Autism

So what *can* be determined at each early age and with what degree of certainty? Here's a brief summary of what can reliably be determined (and what can't, and why) before a child is two, to give you an idea of what any screening done before that age might be worth. If your child is under age two right now, I've also given a few tips on what you can be doing while you wait for a clearer picture to emerge.

Six Months

I've had an opportunity to watch many home movies of children with autism that were made when they were six months old. Even knowing that the child in question will be clearly autistic just two years later, it can be a stretch to point to anything really wrong. Many babies this age (autistic or not) don't look like Mr. Personality when postured for a camcorder and don't seem that alert—they're so busy growing physically that they have little energy left for anything else. Even with a baby who looks outright floppy, unable to track moving objects, or hard to get a (positive or negative) reaction from, even when tickled or bounced, my first thought would not be autism but perhaps moderate to severe mental retardation. In any case, there is not much in the way of interventions that will be useful later that would be useful now. If you're worried about a six-month-old, spend a bit of extra time talking to this baby, having face-to-face contact, and physically engaging the baby (clapping hands and feet, playing peek-a-boo) to alert your baby to his social world.

Twelve Months

In their first-birthday videos, babies who later develop autism often appear frightened or overwhelmed by all the fuss and don't seem to get that this is about them—but neither do shy, anxious, and slow-to-warm babies. It is, however, at this age that we begin to look for several things to appear together that may later become clarified in a diagnosis of autism—not paying attention socially, being in their own world when others try to reach them, and not looking at what you try to get them to look at. More on those signs later in this chapter. If you've seen these signs but your pediatrician says it's too soon to screen, look for your local Early Start agency and take the baby there. In some locales, Early Start services are offered by Easter Seals, UCP (United Cerebral Palsy), ARC (Association for Retarded Citizens), Scottish Rite, Elks, or Shriners' programs, or local departments of public health or developmental disabilities. Your pediatrician should be able to give you this contact information—even if this doctor does not share your concerns at this point. Early Start is a federally mandated avenue for providing help to children birth through age three who are at risk developmentally. Assessors at an Early Start agency will have seen many one-year-olds with a variety of difficulties and will be able to use screening tests at least to rule in or rule out a reason for concern. If there are any Early Start concerns, even at-risk infants and toddlers can be offered services, possibly including a specialized Mommy and Me social group to give you ideas about stimulating your baby, or home visiting where a home visitor can model play with the baby and show you what toys are good and perhaps not so good for development.

In babies we first see at age one we can pretty much rule out any autism about half the time but continue to monitor the other half for overall delays, language delays, *or* possible autism. At this very early age, any development concerns ultimately may be due to any number of other things.

Eighteen Months

By this age language should be on its way. Even if not ready to say words, the baby should be babbling in a communicative way and using plenty of gestures, facial expressions, and strategies like catching your eye to communicate important needs. The typical baby should be enthralled by toys—though his attention span for new and more challenging toys may still be quite limited (and disappointingly short for parents who have just laid out $100 for an age-appropriate "educational" toy). Toy play at this age should simply reflect aspects of the world the baby experiences (being fed, going night-night, getting hugs and kisses, and watching vehicles "go"). With the onset of walking, using parents as a secure base from which to explore becomes quite prominent and casts into relief the social importance of the parents. The baby who "never looks back" at this stage is more worrisome, as even very independent babies will look back to parents for information, if not just security.

Twenty-Four Months

By age two, if a child is still not talking, her social differences from friends' babies are pretty noticeable, and she doesn't play like other children, you definitely should be concerned. At two, this is true even for the baby who doesn't spend much time around other infants and toddlers. If you've been told that two is "too young" to tell, know that this is inaccurate. On the other hand, if you haven't gotten to a specialist until your child is two because you've had to wait months for appointments for various assessments—like speech or occupational therapy (which, by the way, can certainly be scheduled at the same time as an autism assessment)—or you just haven't been sure that something was wrong, don't despair. Concerns at two years of age are not to be ignored, *but it is still quite early enough to achieve the best treatment outcome.*

There are reasons why it's difficult to be certain that a child has autism before one and a half or two years, which will help you remember why a screening test, especially one done at a young age, is never definitive.

Key Screening Concept: Specificity

The younger a child is, the more *nonspecific* his behavior is. Let's start with newborns, who have the greatest amount of *nonspecific* behavior. All a distressed newborn can do is cry. It might mean he's wet, hungry, even sick—or just wanting to be held. We therefore say that crying in a newborn is *nonspecific.* By the time a typically developing child is age three, he can say that he needs to go potty, that he wants apple juice, that his tummy hurts, or "Mommy, pick me up!" He can get *real* specific. This means that the earlier you try to screen for autism, the more nonspecific the things you observe will be—and the problem might just as well be something else or nothing. *Specificity* is a measure of how unique a behavior is to the disorder in which it occurs.

This brings us to the second point: The way we improve "specificity" is to have a detailed understanding of the *qualities* of the behavior we are examining. A good example in the case of autism is early attachment behavior. Although it was questioned in the past, children with autism *are* notably attached to their parents, but the *qualities* of their attachment behaviors are very different from what's normally expected: A child with autism may cry bitterly upon separation from a parent but then seem barely to react when the parent soon thereafter reenters the house or room. In a typically developing eighteen-month-old (as compared to one with autism), a bitter separation response would quickly be followed by a rush up to the parent, clinging to the parent, and at least a short period where the child could be expected to seek reassurance from being picked up, talked to, looked at, or all three. In an eighteen-month-old with autism, the reunion of parent and child is often quite casual. It might consist of the parent having to approach the child and then the child getting soothed by being draped over the parent's legs or tossed over the parent's shoulders like a sack of potatoes. The child would likely not cling (or even "mold") and most often would not seek out the parent's face for reassurance.

Delayed versus Atypical

The image that the general public often has of autism involves what we call *atypical signs*—odd behaviors like staring at fingers or flapping fingers and hands when excited. If you based your own concerns on the presence or absence of atypical behavior, however, you might be misled. First of all, there's not much specificity in these atypical signs at an early age. Behavior like hand flapping is not entirely atypical for a nine-month-old (though it is for a two-and-a-half-year-old). Also, all that flaps is not autism. We also know, for instance, that many perfectly well-developed siblings of children with autism may go through a pro-longed flapping (or toe-walking) phase. These two facts make it diffi-cult for parents to use "atypical" behavior to judge whether something different and worrisome is going on.

Most of the early signs of autism can be characterized as things the child has not yet begun to do—like talk, be as interested in other babies as you might think your baby should be, hug dollies, and so on. That is, the early signs of autism are better characterized as delays than as anything atypical. But how do you tell what is "just" a delay from au-tism? The best way to know there might be a real problem by age two is to look for signs of what is called "the triad of social impairments." This means that the child is having across-the-board difficulties or de-lays in the skills needed for social attention, communication, and play with toys and objects.

Autism Is Many Things at Once

By focusing on the *synchronicity* among lines of development, we learn a great deal about whether some atypical pattern of development may be emerging. *Synchronicity*, in this case, refers to whether social devel-opment, receptive and expressive language development, problem solving, and fine and gross motor development are all pretty much coming along at the same rate—or whether, as in the case of autism spectrum disorders, social and language understanding in particular may be progressing more slowly. Autism is, at its core, a social disabil-ity. A child who is language delayed but socially stronger (where lan-guage is not involved) is not likely autistic.

Autism is many things at once. Just like the expression "One swallow does not make a springtime," one situation where a baby avoids peers, one type of toy a baby refuses to touch, and certain people a baby refuses to acknowledge do not make her autistic. It is only when many of these difficulties exist to some extent simultaneously and across various situations that there is reason for concern. Ask yourself whether the screening for your child has taken that into account.

Specific Qualities That Screening Should Take into Account

When you get together a whole list of behaviors with autism-specific qualities, like the issue of unusual reunions after separation, they outline a map of the child's unique difficulties. If there are enough concerns, the child is said to screen "positive" for autism. It's always important to have a screener with items that form a coherent picture, so you know the positive screen is not just likely reflecting your anxiously completing a screening questionnaire in search of an answer—any answer. In assessing whether a child screens positive for autism, it is important to consider the quality of the behavior of concern—not just whether the child does something yet. Not only does quality matter, but quantity matters too. If a cranky, tired, or angry child very occasionally greets you with an "autistic" reunion, it just may be that he is cranky, tired, or angry. This means that after you complete an autism screener, it is really very important for a professional who knows lots of children with autism to judge whether the qualities and quantities (or threshold) rise to the level where we should be concerned about autism. This is why it is so difficult for you to accurately screen your child for autism on your own. These days we see many parents of first or only children, or older or working parents, who are uncertain about what to expect in their child's development because they really have little chance to see other babies to learn what is absolutely typical at different early ages.

With the PDDST-II screening test for autism, I've included a glossary for the professional who has given the PDDST-II to the parent to complete. This person, even a pediatrician with no special knowledge of autism or developmental disabilities, can then ask more specific questions and ascertain whether a parent's concerns do indeed rise to the level of significant concern about autism.

Is this what occurred when your child was screened? It's likely you'll feel more comfortable with the results of any screening if you're asked thoughtful questions that delve into the quality and quantity of the signs and symptoms at the core of your worries. If you're fortu-

---

Early Concerns That May Indicate a Very Young Child Has Autism

- Bored by conversations around him
- Seemingly uninterested in talking or babbling to communicate
- Actively avoids social situations
- Alert to some sounds, not others
- Interested in (repetitive) motion more than others the same age
- Likes tickles and chasing but not patty cake or peek-a-boo
- Doesn't point, follow a point, or look to see if you see what he's looking at

---

nate, an autism-savvy pediatrician may be listening for you to describe concerns that form the triad of social impairments—in language, social interaction, and play—mentioned earlier.

"He's Not Talking"

The single best early screening item for autism on the PDDST-II is a positive response to the question "Does your baby ever seem bored or uninterested in conversations around him?" The baby who seems not to pay attention to adults talking (as if trying to "learn the language"), who does not seem to follow conversation by looking back and forth between speakers, who does not seem to mirror the marked facial expression of a speaker who suddenly giggles, laughs out loud, or seems about to cry may be autistic. Now please, be certain, I am not saying that babies can be expected to follow all adult conversation like you might follow the batter and pitcher when bases are loaded at the bottom of the third inning with two outs and two strikes. However, the baby who virtually never attends to the main social "action" around him is one who has begun to create that autistic impression of being in "his own little world."

"She Doesn't Play with Toys"

What should you be paying attention to besides the baby's ability to focus social attention? Another big area is playfulness. Babies are not taught to hug dolls or stuffed animals, nor to pretend with their "small world" toys (like a plastic cell phone or a teacup). In the second half of the first year of life, babies cuddle animate toys and in the first half of the second year reenact behavior they see others perform. Again, this is not an all-or-nothing proposition. It's not uncommon for boys to eschew stuffed animals in favor of trucks and cars. However, if this play starts to take on a circumscribed, attenuated quality—playing with only one part of the toy, like the wheels, or doing only one thing with the toy, like lining it up with others, we know there is more reason for concern. It can be hard for a parent to see the boundary between play that is typical and behavior that is not: Many toys these days come in sets—dinos, army men, Matchbox cars—and there is a certain functionality in lining them up. It's when lining things up is the only thing that child does, or when he will line up everything and anything, that there might be real cause for concern. Do know, however, that typically developing children will sometimes line up toys or use them repetitively in the early years.

"He Doesn't Play with Others"

A third area is peer interest. Again, finding other kids interesting is not something babies have to be taught. By that second half of the first year, two crawling babies put on the floor with one another will probably check each other out. They may have no skill at doing this and may grab the other baby by the hair or fingers—but the interest is there. Babies this age don't need to be with others to develop this kind of interest—and often they can't make much of time with another baby either—but the initial interest should be apparent. The baby who actively escapes such situations or seems to form a little "force field" around herself is the baby to be concerned about.

"Isn't It Odd for a Baby to Do That?"

Even though early on, delays are considered more indicative of autism than atypical behavior, actions like posturing fingers, staring at them, or gazing sideways at objects will be considered in a screening and should be reported to the doctor. As discussed earlier, some children line toys up rather than using them in the intended (and, one would think, more compelling) manner. Others become interested in a line of alphabet blocks at age one, and still are just as fascinated at age two, even though they still wouldn't give Elmo or Winnie-the-Pooh a second glance. When a child may have autism, there can be a sense that the child's attention and what she finds of most interest are all mixed up for a child that age.

An Absence of Joint Attention Is a Fundamental Concern

In all of the situations just described, there also is one overarching quality that is likely the most important indicator of whether we should have concerns about autism. This is something called "joint attention"—what occurs when the baby checks in with his mother (looks at her, reaches for her) as if to say "What's happening here? Is this okay?" This is the core instinctive organizing behavior that allows a baby to create a social world. The baby who does not look at his mother as she converses, does not look at his father as his truck makes a great sound, and does not look for help when he has been grabbed by another baby may lack an essential social ingredient that is an early sign of a capacity to form a social world: namely the idea that parents can "read his mind," which the twelve- to fifteen-month-old baby should be able to verify with just a questioning look in a critical situation. We are not talking about unbroken eye contact here, but rather the ability to read a parent when there is a question.

The Screening Results

If your child has screened positive, you will need to start looking for sources of diagnostic assessment. If your child has screened "negative" for autism—or your pediatrician has downplayed your concerns and discouraged you from getting a screening—what do you do?

As far as I know, no one has explicitly studied this, but pediatricians seem to have a bias toward seeing physically well-developed children as developmentally well developed. If a baby is an ex-preemie, has mild CP (cerebral palsy), or has a minor birth defect (like two fused toes), it seems pediatricians are much more alert to the possibility of developmental problems in that child. In autism, there are no consistently associated findings such as these, and perhaps this is one reason autism is so often missed. This is another reason to be prepared with a well-documented list of your concerns ahead of time when you are screened or rescreened by your child's pediatrician.

You know—we certainly do—that if you have older typically developing children, you'll notice the difference between your older children and one who doesn't seem to be following the same path. So don't be too quick to accept a pediatrician's reassurances if you're quite sure you're seeing something different with this child—especially if what you see fits with the list on page 20. If, on the other hand, you have an older child with autism, you've probably been watching the younger sibling with eagle eyes. Most babies seen for possible autism at around a year of age are younger siblings of children already known to have autism. Even if you can see that the younger sibling seems fine early on, as most parents can, you may not be sure enough to dismiss this possibility on your own. The likelihood of a child with autism having a brother or sister with autism is only one in about thirty-three to fifty, but as many as one in four siblings of children with autism may have some minor difficulty like a language delay or being socially just a little standoffish. These signs may heighten your concern unnecessarily. You may in fact be seeing early signs of something that ultimately is not on the autism spectrum but might require a little speech therapy or an extra year of kindergarten. But try to keep this in perspective. If your early observations have told you this child doesn't have the problems his older brother or sister had at that age, screening that rules out concerns about autism may very well be accurate.

Where to Go after Screening "Positive"

One possibility that I haven't raised, which I've seen in about 10% or so of the families I meet, is the astute, well-trained pediatrician who has learned a thing or two about development along the way and raises concerns about autism in your child before you do. If you have a doctor like this, ask her to tell you exactly what gives her that impression. See if those concerns line up with the checklist or other things you've read earlier in this chapter, and if they do, beseech your pediatrician to help you get your child in for further specialized assessment soon.

After a child has screened positive for autism, it's time to start looking for further assessment that can lead to a diagnosis and a treatment plan. There are a couple ways to go. In the past, before autism screeners were available to pediatricians, and before pediatricians had increased awareness of developmental disabilities, a child referred beyond primary pediatric care for developmental assessment might spend six to twelve months (when he could be in treatment) just going through the diagnostic "pipeline." This was because pediatricians would often want to obtain "rule-out" testing first.

What Is "Rule-Out" Testing?

Rule-out tests are those that the doctor may order to make sure the child's problems are *not* due to some condition that may not be seen. Rule-outs are especially called for if there is some suspicious sign, like not responding to sound, neurological soft signs (atypical motor development or absence of muscle reflexes a pediatrician regularly tests), or minor congenital anomalies (unusual birthmarks, tags of skin, any malformation). But the important thing to know about rule-out tests is that *if your child has screened positive for autism, he should go straight to an autism assessment*—even if the rule-out testing is also to be scheduled. This ensures that the child can get treatment as soon as possible.

"How Can I Be Sure My Child Hears If He Doesn't Answer?"

For children who might be autistic, the most common kind of rule-out testing ordered by pediatricians is testing to rule out a hearing loss as the reason that the child seems not to be responsive to speech and not talking himself. It is always important to go through such testing if hearing might be compromised, and especially important to do so sooner rather than later if the baby already has a history of recurrent ear infections or tubes to drain fluid from his ears. It is usually clear to parents of toddlers with autism that their child *can* hear. While he might turn and respond to his name only 50% of the time, he may always run to the TV when he hears the *Teletubbies* theme music. This is not a child with a hearing loss so significant that he cannot develop speech. It is something else, and it is quite possibly autism.

Neurological, Genetic, and Metabolic Testing

Similarly, a pediatrician may want to obtain neurological, genetic, or metabolic testing for a child who may have autism. The first thing for a parent to know is that most children with autism will not have any positive findings when seen by a neurologist. Most kinds of brain measurements are normal in children with autism, though research does suggest subtle architectural differences in brain structure that cannot be picked up in clinical tests using MRI, CT, MEG, EEG (magnetic resonance imaging, computed tomography, magnetoencephalography, electroencephalography), and the like. Further, unless a child has a seizure disorder, there is no treatment for any neurological abnormality that might be found in the structure of the brain. If a child has seizures, parents usually suspect them. Only a tiny number of children with autism have seizures (other than febrile seizures) at the age they are when they are being worked up for an autism diagnosis.

Another area for possible rule-out workup is karyotyping—looking at the child's chromosomes to make sure they are all there, correctly formed, and there are not too many (like in Down syndrome). While many genetic abnormalities have been associated with a small subset of cases in autism, there are no specific treatments based on these. Mainly, the genetic testing is of most urgent interest to parents thinking of having another child sometime soon. Some pediatricians do not recommend a full karyotyping but do recommend testing for fragile X syndrome—once thought to be much more strongly associated with autism (and now understood to be present in about only half a percent of all cases of autism).

"Level 2" Developmental Testing: Seeing a Doctor Who Can Say Whether It's Autism or Not

Once parent and pediatrician agree that there is concern about autism, it's time to select the type of further testing that will be most helpful in identifying services the child needs. There are basically two ways to go: One is to proceed to what is sometimes called "Level 2" assessment, meaning the child is being specifically assessed for any developmental problems that are present. The other way to proceed is to go straight to an autism-specific assessment.

Many centers that provide "Level 2"-type assessments, such as hospital child development centers, special education intake units, or assessment units for departments of public health or developmental disabilities are equipped with a team of staff that can be deployed as needed to administer tests specifically designed for characterizing different specific problems including autism. These more generalist settings may be where you need to go first because (1) that is what your health insurance covers, (2) you need to qualify for services, or (3) there are no autism-specific clinics in your area. These places are particularly good settings for assessment if there are some significant "differential diagnosis" questions. ("Differential diagnoses" are the other conditions the doctor will consider as alternative or additional explanations for your child's difficulties.) This means that if a severe language impairment, moderate to severe mental retardation, attention deficit disorder, or behavioral problems have also been suggested as a reason for your child's difficulties, you may be better off starting at a place with clinicians experienced at identifying any of these as well as autism.

If you have a choice of where to go for assessment right after screening positive for possible autism with your pediatrician, and there are no really worrisome differential diagnoses, you should go straight to an autism-specific clinic where clinicians use autism-specific measures to identify aspects of your child's specific difficulties that can then be mapped directly onto different treatment approaches. If your pediatrician is one who has used a specific autism screening test like the PDDST-II with you, she likely knows the resources for evaluating a child for autism that exist in your locale. If not, your local department of developmental services or public health can provide either a clinic or referral to such a clinic. Many pediatricians these days are bound to referring you to a "Level 2" evaluator within your HMO, PPO, or "network." You may want to check whether this person is really experienced at autism assessment or just happens to have signed up for that "panel." When you call this clinician's office, you can ask what conditions other than autism this clinician sees for assessment, how many cases of autism are assessed each year, and whether the assessment will include a treatment plan. I would recommend trying to find a diagnostician for whom autism spectrum disorders are 25% or more of the assessments he or she does each year.

Moving On to Diagnostic Assessment

This chapter should have helped you determine whether any screening you've already gotten was conducted systematically and the results seem accurate. If not, you have a road map to follow for having your child screened again. If you're now convinced that your child needs a comprehensive assessment, you'll want to learn exactly what this entails so that you can ensure that the assessment you obtain or have obtained for your child has "the right stuff." This means more than a label. But, what if you feel like all you're ending up with *is* a label? Do you need a label at all? What components should you look for in a comprehensive assessment? How long will it take? How do you get assessors and "treaters" communicating with one another? The next chapter will help you answer these questions.

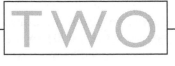

Getting Your Footing

WHAT A DIAGNOSIS CAN (AND SHOULD) DO FOR YOU AND YOUR CHILD

In this chapter and the next, we'll focus on all the specific things you need to know to make sure your child's evaluation and diagnosis have done what they're supposed to do—point you as directly as possible to a comprehensive treatment plan. Here we'll start with the whole question of labeling: Does your child need to be labeled with a particular autism spectrum disorder to get the services that will help? Then I'll describe exactly what the ideal diagnostic evaluation looks like—the set of procedures that have proven most likely to lead to that customized treatment plan you want. Although you'll have to be somewhat flexible to acknowledge realities such as what facilities and experts are accessible to you, it's this "best-practice" diagnosis that should be your goal.

   If the assessments and specific tests described in the following pages are all familiar to you, you can probably take heart that you've already gotten a comprehensive evaluation. But if you spot gaps, you might want to talk to your doctor about whether your child's evaluation has truly been adequate without these pieces. And, of course, if your child hasn't yet been assessed, you can use the information here as a roadmap to get what you need at the outset.

Why Do We Need a Diagnostic Label?

Diagnostic Signs as a Shorthand for Treatment Needs

When you say that a child has autism, you mean that he needs to acquire some social skills, learn to improve his communicative use of language, and play more like other children his age. In this sense the diagnostic label is a shorthand for treatment needs. This label does not tell us whether a particular child given the label can talk at all, has behavior problems that interfere with the ability to learn, or is also mentally retarded and will learn more slowly than a child who is not. The diagnostic *process*, however, *can* tell us that and a lot more.

Treatment programs for children with autism usually incorporate features that are tailored to the learning strengths and weaknesses of a child with autism: Such programs tend to emphasize visual supports to help the child process auditory (heard) information, special reinforcement strategies that motivate, and ways of incrementally developing social interaction skill. However, not all children diagnosed with an autism spectrum disorder need every one of these (and other) special features in their treatment plan; it will depend on which symptoms of autism they have. A big goal of going through the diagnostic process with your child, then, is to learn which of these autistic-type learning difficulties she has and what autism-specific treatment strategies are available to address them. This means that some children on the autistic spectrum will need to be in programs designed specifically for children with autism, while others can be accommodated in more mainstreamed settings that are individually designed to meet special needs as well as foster areas of development that may be basically okay—at or around age expectations.

The diagnosis ("label") of autism or a related autism spectrum disorder *is* often the "ticket" a child needs for admission into specific special educational services. To the extent that the diagnostic label fits, the child *will* need some of these services. In this chapter and Chapter 3 we're focusing on what the diagnostic assessment should look like. In Part III of this book we'll tackle the much more complex task of teaching you how to figure out how your individual child learns and then which programs and features of programs will likely be most effective.

Are More Things Being Called "Autism"?

Another dimension to understand (ideally as you move into the diagnostic process but certainly by the time you emerge from it) is how the diagnosis of autism has expanded—everywhere from doctors' offices, to schools, to reports in the media. In the Introduction to this book, I said I would be using the word *autism* as shorthand for *autism spectrum disorders* but that all the issues and principles we would cover would have relevance whether your child had been given a diagnosis of autistic disorder, pervasive developmental disorder not otherwise specified (PDDNOS), or Asperger syndrome (or disorder).

Autism has only recently been thought of as a "spectrum disorder." What does *spectrum disorder* imply anyway? By *spectrum* we really mean two things: One, some children will have more of the symptoms associated with all twelve of the diagnostic criteria for autism (shown in Chapter 3) than others. Two, some children will have more severe symptoms than others. We also have mental retardation cutting across this spectrum, adding another dimension. As autism has increasingly been recognized as a spectrum disorder, more children who were formerly characterized as autistic-like or having autistic features or being language-impaired and socially aloof are increasingly seen as "on the spectrum." This is because the symptoms of autism are ubiquitous. No single symptom of autism occurs only in autism. Children with language disorders can be echolalic (repeating words or phrases or fragments of them unexpectedly). Mentally retarded children can have motor stereotypies (like toe walking and repetitively flexing wrists or fingers). Children with anxiety disorders can be very prone to avoiding peers.

If a child has the same symptoms as a child with autism, will that child require the same help that an autistic child will need to overcome the same difficulty? Maybe; maybe not. Any good treatment plan that comes from a good diagnostic assessment will consider each individual child's weaknesses *and* strengths. When the symptom is the same but the diagnosis is different, the two children with the same weakness but different diagnoses will have different relative strengths with which to overcome the weakness—which means they will need to be taught differently. For example, if a child avoids peers because he is anxious, he is likely to have a different pattern of social strengths (like being very dependent on cues from his mother) than a child who actually has autism.

This is why, from a treatment point of view, getting a diagnosis "on the spectrum" for having any symptom of autism—without considering it in the context of other strengths and weaknesses—can cause tremendous confusion when planning treatment and later, when treatment starts.

Where on the spectrum a child is diagnostically does not alone inform us about needed treatments either, because the spectrum is multidimensional—cognitively high versus cognitively low; verbal versus nonverbal; behaviorally challenged versus passive, and so on. When we ignore where a child is on the spectrum, unhelpful educational treatment can result: Sometimes a high-functioning child with an autism spectrum disorder is offered services for low-functioning children and is put into a class where he is the only child with spoken language ability. In other places, low-functioning children with autism spectrum disorders are mainstreamed with only a recently trained aide because such an approach has "worked" with higher-functioning children with autism spectrum disorders at that school. What all this can add up to is that the autism spectrum disorder "label" can be very helpful when it gets you in the door to service. *You as the parents will just have to be vigilant to see it's the right door.*

One thing that you'll learn along the road to getting help for your child with autism is that there seems to be so much more autism than there once was. Aside from the emergence of the concept of autism as a spectrum disorder, there are several reasons for reports of increased incidence, and it's beyond the scope of this book to go into all of them. From the point of view of a parent seeking services, though, the oft-reported increase in autism is a double-edged sword. On one hand, as incidence has risen, so has the number of autism-specific services available. On the other hand, these services tend to be expensive because they require special training and intensive staffing ratios, so educational authorities understandably mete out such resources very judiciously. Many parents hear of these services, naturally want to try them, and then are frustrated trying to get them. A more efficient approach than trying anything and everything is to focus your efforts on getting what will really help *your* child. This book will help you do that by teaching you to figure out what your child needs. When new treatment options keeping cropping up, as the following brief history shows, knowing specifically what your child needs is a better way to know which advances to take advantage of than just jumping on the latest better-built mousetrap because someone else—even an expert—says it's the way to help children with autism.

A (Very) Brief History of the Diagnosis and Treatment of Autism

Twenty years ago, most children with autism were served in classes alongside other children with comparable levels of disability. This meant that severely retarded autistic children were placed with other severely retarded children. Period. More "medium"-functioning children with autism would be in classes with more mildly to moderately retarded children. Period. Either what we now regard as high-functioning autism was not identified with an autism diagnosis or such children were placed in classes for children with communicative impairments—though these children had more trouble knowing *when* to talk (pragmatics) than *how* to talk (semantics). Children who are now designated as having Asperger syndrome were seldom recognized as having an autism diagnosis (expect perhaps in the first few years of life) and either received no special services or got some patchwork of private services and therapies their parents would cobble together on an ad hoc basis.

If we go back more than thirty years, to before 1975 and the first federal law guaranteeing special education to all children, there were fewer programs still. Poorer and more impaired children might receive day treatment of a vaguely educational nature through residential public institutions (the first setting in which I learned to work with children with autism). If the children came from very well-off families, they would be sent to handsome residential schools in lovely rural settings (but with curricula similar to what children in the public hospitals received). (This was the second type of setting in which I worked for children with autism.) In those days, the early 1970s, autism was just emerging from the dark shadow of psychoanalytic treatment. We understood that psychodynamic treatment (in which the therapist and patient work together to uncover unconscious, unresolved conflicts from the past as a way to explain the patient's current symptoms) was a futile approach for autism—but we did not yet know what else to do.

In the 1980s, treatment approaches such as the work instigated by the late Dr. Eric Schopler at Project TEACCH in North Carolina initiated the use of strong routines, high predictability, and strong visual supports, playing to the strengths of the autistic learner. It was a big breakthrough and the first time we had an autism-specific curriculum.

In the late 1980s, Dr. Ivar Lovaas at UCLA published a paper showing how principles of behavior modification (developed mainly on rats and pigeons and the like) could be applied to children with autism using a codified behavioral methodology called *discrete trial training* (DTT). Using an experimentally controlled curriculum, he showed remarkable improvements to more children with autism than had ever been successfully treated before. The conceptual shift that Dr. Lovaas introduced was another breakthrough.

Standards for Autism Treatment Today

In the last fifteen years, Lovaas's work has not been fully replicated, but it is now generally accepted that behavioral methods, including discrete trial training, are powerful tools in treating autism. The original models offered by both Schopler and Lovaas have been taken up by many others and modified and refined in ways that give us a much broader range of tools for autistic children of different ages and at different levels of functioning. Many others have innovated treatments for autism as well, which has further expanded the repertoire for teachers and therapists working with children with autism.

If you're just starting to grapple with how to get your child treated, this brief history is meant to offer a couple of succinct lessons: The first is that the field of autism treatment is always growing and changing; new ideas that may be worth exploring for your child will always be emerging. Second, what a child is "entitled" to as part of special education is the result of a complex and changing (and, to some extent, local) formula of what methods and services have been put in place. What any one child "gets" is likely to be a result of not only what is prescribed in treatment plans made by assessors but also what is available, what parents know about and ask for, and what other children in the same school jurisdiction have gotten (or not gotten). Treatment standards are constantly being modified as new practices are introduced for one child and, if successful, become available to others.

Special Issues for Parents of Children with High-Functioning Autism

Increasingly, as autism is understood to be a "spectrum" disorder, we realize there are many children who have a full or partial "phenotype." This means that many individuals have some or all of the genes involved with autism and that some or all of these genes may be strongly enough expressed to cause adaptive difficulties. Since children get their genes from parents, parents too may have a few forms of some of the traits of autism, or a mild version of them. Some of these traits can be quite beneficial—like having a "math" brain, being quite dogged and persistent at a task once it is undertaken, and needing any job worth doing to be done well. This is not to say that any parent of a child with autism who is smart, works hard, or cares about the quality of his or her work product is being a bit autistic for being that way. It becomes a diagnosis only if it occurs to such a maladaptive degree that the individual cannot carry out the full range of tasks needed for daily living. At the preschool level, these tasks include getting along with peers and wanting to follow directions. In an adult they include communicating effectively with coworkers and understanding what a manager at work expects from you.

At what point do these traits become a problem that needs treatment? How do you know whether shades of these traits that you see in your child actually rise to the level of a "diagnosis"? When do they rise to the level of a diagnosis that will benefit from treatments specifically designed for children with autism? When your child's quirkiness, "geekiness," or obsessiveness begins to limit where he can go, define who he can be with, and whether peers avoid him, these eccentricities have become maladaptive in his world. That's when it's time to get a professional opinion.

If You're Hesitant to "Label" Your High-Functioning/Asperger Syndrome Child

One issue I am often asked about is whether a child's teachers or therapist need to be told the child is "on the spectrum" or actually has autism. As I've argued so far, getting the diagnosis will be the single most helpful step in opening the door to a range of services. When the "label" qualifies the higher-functioning child for school services, it will be difficult for professionals associated with the school not to be aware of the child's qualifying condition. However, when it comes to preschools, after-school programs, recreation programs, and private schools, parents may have more of a choice. These are the issues: If your child is likely to need special supports such as an aide accompanying him, it will be obvious to everyone that he has *something*, and it will be natural for them to start to figure it out right away. If you offer a subterfuge like saying, "Well, he's young and I want him to have extra help because I realize he's not as mature as others his age," no one will be fooled for a moment. Those involved in such programs will likely either hint or demand that your child be assessed, telling you that it could be "more" than immaturity. If they can see your child has a problem, and think you know too, an honest and open relationship with people you are expecting to teach and help your child will work best all around.

Strategies for Inclusion That Avoid Labeling

Some children, though, can be passed off as something other than on the autism spectrum. Among the highest-functioning 10% or so, this is often an important consideration for parents. An aide can be supplied because the child "has severe language-processing problems" or "a central auditory processing disorder" or has been language delayed and "can understand but still doesn't really talk much." Since many adults in non-autism-specific treatment settings are familiar with only the "average" autistic child—who may be much more severely disabled than your child—this alternative labeling explains why it might be difficult for the child to participate fully at times but also helps prevent overly low expectations. In these situations, you can consider using your child's diagnosis on a need-to-know basis, telling when asked or when it becomes clear that your child will need further adaptations to the learning environment.

The potential "cost" of disclosing your child's diagnosis when it really does not need to be known is in stigma alone. When parents of typically developing children hear "autism" or "Asperger," they may become overly solicitous—or unfriendly. Other children may "mascot" your child, including her but only as they would a much younger sibling, relegating her to only low expectations to be lived up to (or down to).

Saying the Emperor Has Clothes Doesn't Make It So

Most parents don't find themselves with a very high-functioning child when autism has been diagnosed, and rarely in the first years of treatment. For you, then, the decision about whether to reveal your child's diagnosis may have to be based on other considerations. For some parents the diagnosis provides relief—that these problems have a name, that there are things to be done, that there are other children and other families facing the same thing. But, quite understandably, not everyone is ready to become a member of the "club" right away. If you're in this group, reading things like this book can ameliorate the feeling that your child now has a "label" by letting you see that allying yourself with sources of information about autism is instrumentally helpful. So can adhering to the spirit of the politically correct child-first syntax that favors the term *child with autism* over *autistic child*. Taking this language to heart is a way of acknowledging that your child is indeed your child first and that "autistic" is just one part of your son or daughter.

However, avoiding the label in an "emperor has no clothes" attempt to deny the diagnosis out of existence tends not to work either. This obfuscation just closes the door on the open, collaborative, honest dialogue that will always be needed between parents and their child's treaters.

Getting a "Best-Practice" Diagnosis

So now you know why you need a diagnosis: The diagnosis opens the door to services, and the diagnosis is a shorthand for many, but not all, treatment needs. The diagnostic assessment should help you understand specifically what's wrong with your child in particular. If you've already had an assessment done, and it hasn't provided this understanding, you can use this chapter to identify what *wasn't* included in your child's evaluation so you can go back and fill in the gaps. So far you should know that because autism is a "spectrum" disorder, your child won't necessarily be labeled as simply autistic or not. Your child may have been found to be "fully" autistic and may have gotten a diagnosis of "autistic disorder." Or she could be said to have a "partial" autistic syndrome and get a diagnosis of PDDNOS or Asperger syndrome. You could be told as part of the diagnostic assessment that your child has some "autistic traits" that might be addressed productively with treatments designed mainly for children with autism. If so, know that some people will say your child is "on the spectrum" and others will not, but that's not really the important thing. The important thing for you will be to learn whether there are treatments designed for children with autism from which your child may benefit. If there are such treatments, how should you set out to get them?

The next part of this chapter explains how children with autism need to be assessed so that you can have confidence that any diagnosis your child receives or has received is correct. A "best-practice" diagnosis means, essentially, one based on everything known in the field to lead to the best possible outcome for the child. Even more important, I'll explain how the diagnostic assessment process should help you understand what treatments your child needs and why.

Why a Comprehensive Assessment Is Best

By "comprehensive," we mean an assessment that looks at many aspects of the child's behavior and abilities. This approach allows for a full appraisal of strengths and weaknesses so that the former can be used to compensate for the latter in the treatment plan. For children, especially very young children, the child's level of development must be taken into account too, because it points the way to what skills need to be established next.

All Roads Lead to Rome: Basing a Diagnosis on Multiple Traits, Using Multiple Methods

If you were going to buy a car, you might list the things you wanted in a new car down the left side of a spreadsheet. Across the top, you might list four or five cars that interested you. Then you'd fill in the spreadsheet with "yes"s and "no"s to indicate which cars had which desirable qualities. If you were completely rational, you'd then buy the car topping the column with the most "yes"s. Many paths would have led you to the same answer to the question "What car shall I buy?" This is what we call *convergent validity*, and we look for it when we assess a child for autism. We look at many traits of the child. We look at each trait in different ways. A child who was observed to avoid all the other kids in a doctor's waiting room may have a screaming great time with his cousins in his own home. The doctor who concludes your child "lacks peer relations" because your child does not like to be around new kids in a new place does not have all the data points he needs.

Assessing Symptoms by Looking at Multiple Traits

The best way to carry out a comprehensive assessment, therefore, is to measure each possible symptom of autism in multiple ways. One questionnaire, one answer to one question, one example is not enough to demonstrate that a particular symptom of autism is present. Why? One of the twelve diagnostic criteria for autism is having a "lack of varied, spontaneous make-believe play or social imitative play appropriate to developmental level."* A child who repeatedly lines up toys and then does little else with them is often considered to meet this criterion. But if the child just so happens to be a three-year-old boy who loves Thomas the Tank Engine and endlessly puts Thomas on and off the track, gazing at his wheels, rolling him back and forth only slightly, it might be autism or it might not be. This is what Thomas the Tank Engine is made to do. Most Thomas paraphernalia is not purchased by parents of children with autism. If there were other examples, such as that the child lined up objects not usually lined up—like crayons *and* Legos *and* playing cards—*and* never colored, never built buildings or tried to play Go Fish, I would become increasingly concerned. But even then I'd want more examples—more methods, more ways of measuring this "trait." What else does the child do with toys that seems consistent with a "lack of imagination"? Does he eschew cuddling Winnie-the-Pooh? Has he never fed a baby doll? Has he never pretended Buzz Lightyear can fly? If the child never or rarely did any of these things, then there really is some evidence that the trait in question is present.

	Sources of information (on multiple "methods")			
Multiple traits	**Direct observations (home versus school)**	**Parent reports (mother versus father)**	**Records of earlier assessments and treatments**	**Teacher/ therapist reports**
Social signs and symptoms	X	X	X	X
Communication problems	X	X	X	X
Unusual activities and interests	X	X	X	X

*American Psychiatric Association. (2000). *Diagnostic and statistical manual of mental disorders* (4th ed., text rev.). Washington, DC: Author.

Using Multiple Methods

In addition to having varied examples of each sign of autism, we need to measure each sign in at least some different ways. That way an assessor can be sure the sign is real and not just an artifact of a particular situation or a particular person's way of describing things. The table on page 37 shows what I mean.

Questionnaires

Methods can include parent-reported information from questionnaires, as an example. These can be either take-home questionnaires or ones done in conjunction with an examiner. The screening questionnaires discussed in the last chapter fall into this category, as do questionnaires that specifically assess things like diagnostic symptoms (like the CARS [Childhood Autism Rating Scale], the GARS [Gilliam Autism Rating Scale], and the ASDS [Asperger Syndrome Diagnostic Scale]), language development (like the MCDI [McArthur Communication Development Inventory]), adaptive behaviors (like the SIB [Scale of Independent Behavior]), or school readiness skills. There is no one questionnaire that is the "best" one to use. There is no one questionnaire that can tell the clinician, "Diagnose." A questionnaire is always just one part, one method that can be used as part of a multimethod assessment.

Questionnaires are, unfortunately, limited in validity by their *reliability*. Their reliability is really *your* reliability when you're the informant. Reliability in this context means the degree to which your response reflects what you would say every day for a week if asked the same question, or the answer that would be given if both parents and anyone else who knew the child well had to come to an agreement about each and every question. Being reliable also relates to giving a "valid" answer. Is your "sometimes" the same as the "sometimes" that the person who developed the questionnaire had in mind? Are you tending to overreport to make sure the examiner sees this is really a problem or to ensure you will get services? Are you tending to underreport because you aren't ready to believe that what you observed is a "symptom" of something and not just cute-little-kid behavior? All these kinds of errors occur, not out of malice but just because of human nature. What reporting problems do, though, is add "error" to the questionnaire's score. To get a pattern of response to any questionnaire that is reliable and valid, and as helpful as possible to understanding a diagnosis or a treatment plan, your job will be to respond as truthfully and fully as if you were undergoing an IRS audit. This will be the best way to assure that the examiner will learn all she can about your child.

Interviews

Increasingly, autism assessment has come to rely on a specific kind of questionnaire that is described as "interviewer-mediated." This means that an interviewer specifically trained in autism, and specifically trained to use a particular questionnaire, asks the parents questions and queries for specific examples. Then the interviewer categorizes responses as symptom-positive or symptom-negative and also rates severity—based on his or her experience with other cases of autism. This type of interviewer-mediated questionnaire can get around many of the problems of the simpler parent-report questionnaires just enumerated. The best example of this type of questionnaire is the ADI-R (Autism Diagnostic Interview—Revised), which has become standard as part of a diagnostic battery for research subjects. But even the ADI-R in the hands of an experienced examiner needs to be accompanied by methods that directly assess the child, because parent perceptions are always colored by how experienced the parent is with children, how much he or she already knows about autism, and sometimes even whether the child is in the middle of a particularly rough patch or seeming to be doing much better all of a sudden. The ADI-R can take up to two and a half hours to administer, so most parents will not encounter it as part of a diagnostic assessment for their child unless the clinic happens to be part of a research program. This doesn't mean the assessment was less than A+, but it does mean that some other way of systematically surveying specific symptoms of autism has been used.

More common is the semistructured interview where the assessor has a general list of topics to cover one at a time. In the following chapter, I'll talk about the topics that each type of assessor typically should include in a thorough assessment. However, in many autism or developmental clinics, parents will encounter a "primary clinician" who will take the child's history and get details on each of the twelve specific symptoms of autism. This includes asking questions about the child's social development, her play and imagination, and any odd or unusual interests or behaviors.

A good examiner is one who asks questions about these areas with the child's overall developmental level in mind. For children with autism, chronological age expectations are only part of the picture. The examiner also needs to get an idea of the degree of overall developmental delay, if any, and to adjust expected social behaviors and play milestones accordingly. This should be done as part of the direct assessment of the child.

Observations

Observation should be used as well. It can be informal or "naturalistic" (observations made at a child's home, school, or a clinic), but also can include videotapes of the child in settings the clinical examiner may not otherwise have a chance to assess. (In our clinic, for example, parents are asked to bring brief videos of children at play with peers since we're not going to have a better way to assess this in a clinic.) In a naturalistic observation, the child just plays around. This gives an examiner an opportunity to assess how, on his own, a child makes use of his time and his environment. If you're asked, by the way, not to bring a child's favorite toys to an assessment or into an examining room, it's not that the examiner isn't interested in what your child can do but rather that she is interested in what he *will* do, compared to others under the same circumstances. Conversely, a home or school observation is a chance for a child to be in a familiar place—where behavior may be organized very differently from how it is in a strange new place. All of this is useful information.

Observations can also be semistructured. This means that the assessor has a list of things the child or parent with the child may be asked to do. An example of a semistructured observation would be having the parent step out of the room for a moment and then observing how the child reacts when alone, as well as how the child reacts when the parent comes back in. This type of semistructured observation is a window into the organization of that child's attachment. Important for the examiner, semistructured observations provide an opportunity to compare across children seen under the same conditions. This allows the clinician to make increasingly finer discriminations among the strengths and weaknesses of different children. In our clinic, we use a semistructured observation called the ETHOS, which compares six minutes of the child's play with a parent to six minutes of the child's play with an examiner. Each adult spends two minutes trying to get the child to interact directly without use of any toys, two minutes of ignoring the child and allowing her to play alone and/or observe and join the adult's play, and two minutes of joint adult–child play with what appears to be the child's most preferred toy in the room.

Similarly, structured observations provide an opportunity to create "presses" for certain positive or problematic things to happen. Using the attachment behavior example above, the difference between a structured and a semistructured observation would be if the parent were directed to go back into the room and pick up and cuddle the child, whether or not the child asked for it or seemed to want it. Good standardized structured observations for young children with autism include the STAT (Screening Test for Autism in Toddlers) and the ADOS (Autism Diagnostic Observation Schedule, Module 1). The ADOS also has modules for school-age children and a semistructured interview format for teens and adults with high-functioning autism or Asperger syndrome and was designed as the observational component to complement the ADI-R.

What If Your Child's Assessment Doesn't Include Much Interview or Observation?

A clinician or team who used neither semistructured nor structured assessment is not up to "best-practice" standards. In the olden days, it was acceptable for a doctor to give a diagnosis after fifteen minutes of a little kid running around his office while he chatted with parents. Today it is certainly not. Worse yet is the clinician who tries to play with the child in a medical examining room, or other non-child-friendly environment, and when avoided or rebuffed says, "See—that's autism." The worst example, though, is the clinician who has been known to "diagnose" a child who has slept through the entire assessment—which basically consisted of a chat with a parent in the doctor's study.

If this has happened to you, and you found yourself questioning whether the clinician had an opportunity to see or hear or "feel" the whole story, you are certainly justified in seeking another opinion. If this "look and diagnose" approach turns out to be standard operating procedure for the doctor you have seen, it may not do much good to request that additional methods be used to help you develop a better understanding of your child—because the doctor may not be trained in them. Instead, consider a second opinion. I'd also be concerned that a doctor who conducts cursory diagnostic exams will have a cursory understanding of treatment alternatives—and choosing among those treatments is the ultimate goal of any diagnostic assessment.

Comprehensive = Experts Who Talk to Each Other

So you now understand why assessments must be multitrait, as well as why (and how) they can be designed using multiple methods. Who should you be expecting to carry out this work? Is it better to have your child assessed by one or many people? Simultaneously or in a series of visits? Who has the expertise it takes to diagnose and plan an individualized treatment for a child with autism?

A few years back, I was part of a committee that designed California state standards for assessment of autism. As far as I know, California's Department of Developmental Services is the only state-level agency of its type that has gone so far as to design such specific standards.* These standards were devised because of the incredible rise in the reported incidence of autism in California, the rise in expenditures for autism-related services, and a need to better understand (and standardize) what was getting classified as autism where. In any case, one task we were charged with was producing guidelines that would tie diagnostic assessment to treatment planning via deployment of different kinds of clinicians and different assessment procedures. These standards are what is reflected in the following discussion.

You may have already heard the term *assessment team*. Broadly it can mean either a multidisciplinary team or a transdisciplinary team.

A multidisciplinary team simply is one that includes professionals from many different disciplines—like psychology, psychiatry, education, speech and language, and physical or occupational therapy. In the multidisciplinary team model, each assessor has a circumscribed role. Each examiner sees the child and writes a report. Sometimes the team meets as a group before meeting with parents, and a further comprehensive report that highlights and integrates the findings of the individual reports is also prepared. Then the lead examiner, if there is one, alone or with others from the team, meets with parents and presents the findings, including diagnostic assessment of the child and, hopefully, recommendations for specific, individualized treatment.

This is a very good standard of care, but there are a few assurances you might want to look for or ask for: For one, one or more examiners may have seen the child on a particularly bad day. Another possibility is that in the time between the first part of the assessment and the end you may have started some treatment(s) and seen changes. Did every-

---

*California Department of Developmental Services. (2002). *Autistic spectrum disorders: Best practice guidelines for screening, diagnosis and assessment*. Sacramento, CA: Author.

one on the team know about these? What do they make of the initial treatment response? If there was one clinician you felt connected particularly well with your child, what can you (and the rest of the team) say about those "active ingredients" and what clues for treatment design might they hold? Finally, and most important, if one approach to treatment is being recommended, and you had another in mind, you should certainly ask for the rationale for what *is* being recommended and the "why not" for the one that isn't being recommended. With respect to any nonrecommended treatment, make sure to learn whether the clinician(s) in fact have firsthand knowledge of it. If any of this ground wasn't covered, it would certainly be understandable why you might have misgivings about the diagnosis you received or the treatment recommendations based on it. The point of any assessment is to get you help. If you haven't gotten answers that allow you to understand what can be expected to work (or not) and why—ask more questions.

A transdisciplinary team is one in which professionals from different disciplines work together. This can be a distinct improvement as it removes the "blind men feeling the elephant" hazard. When assessors see the child at different times, under their own conditions, there is a bias for only part of the story to be told or emphasized. In our clinic, for example, one examiner may carry out a language assessment and then another an assessment of nonlanguage intelligence; by itself that's a multidisciplinary setup. However, through a one-way mirror, the other examiner watches, and a supervisor watches too. The child who may have happily whizzed through puzzles, nested cubes, block designs, and mazes may suddenly appear hyperactive, inattentive, and even aggressive if then given a test of receptive or expressive language—with cooperation flagging even as the reinforcement schedule for every bit of on-task behavior is ramped up. If we were just a multidisciplinary team, we might end up with a language examiner who was suggesting a differential diagnosis of attention deficit disorder (ADD) along with a primary diagnosis of autism—while the psychological examiner was left feeling that the child was so cooperative and eager to work that the diagnosis of autism might even seem a bit questionable. Instead, using a transdisciplinary approach, we capture important strengths and weaknesses, and then the team needs to discuss all the data, and the parents need to understand how such information could be integrated into selecting teaching strategies that use strong nonverbal reasoning to help the child decode situations calling for language-based comprehension.

This highlights how critical it is for examiners from each discipline to be aware of and integrate the information their colleagues rely on. When this is not done, you may end up hearing something that does not ring true. You meet with the speech and language pathologist and come away feeling your child has no learning readiness skills. Then you meet with the psychologist who did the nonverbal testing and feel that perhaps you should stop wondering which special education class is best and instead think only about full inclusion. It shouldn't have to be your job to pull everything together on your own. This is all part of good diagnostic assessment and treatment planning.

How Long Does a Good Assessment Take?

To some extent, the length of the assessment has to do with the age of the child. Twenty-month-olds just don't have that much history. Likely nothing in terms of treatment has been tried yet. Likely the baby doesn't talk yet. On the other hand, a twelve-year-old, once thought to be retarded, now thought to be gifted, who once was diagnosed as having ADD but who has had only one friend in his whole life, is going to take a lot longer to assess.

Some teams see the child in one or two intensive days. These assessments are usually done in autism specialty clinics with two or more members of the team present at any one point of the assessment. The advantage of such assessment is that a longer single assessment period gives a chance to see the child before he "warms up," after he does, in a fresh mood, and in a not so fresh mood. The more variability the clinicians can sample, the better. On the other hand, such assessments often do not include a visit to the child's school or to proposed treatment programs or a preliminary home visit to assess how proposed interventions can be best "fitted" to the "ecology" of the family.

Team assessments through developmental service and/or Early Start agencies usually do start with a home visit since a mandate of federal funding is to serve children age zero to three years in their natural environment—usually home. In any case, an infant or toddler is more likely to explore and give the examiner a firsthand demonstration of her activity preferences in her own home.

School assessments tend to get the best look at peer interactions. School-based assessments also have the advantage of affording opportunities where a child (and/or parent) can visit different classes in a search for the best place to implement a treatment plan. When assessment is conducted at school, the "rules of engagement" for the assessment activities closely mirror the rules used for engaging the child in direct instruction—and often the same adults are involved. This can be especially helpful for a school-age child. There is no one right setting or timeline for a diagnostic and treatment planning assessment. Depending on the child's age and the questions being asked, different settings may have different advantages.

Perhaps the only type of assessment to avoid, if possible, is the piecemeal assessment that is protracted over several visits across several weeks. For reasons that are antediluvian and pointless to explain, insurance companies sometimes prefer this model, but I certainly don't. In assessments that involve an hour or two of child assessment and/or parent interview at a time, stretched over four to six weeks, a clinician will have ample opportunity to forget the important things she wanted to tell you about your child, mix him up with someone else, lose paperwork, and put off writing a report till your three-year-old has mentally merged with every other cute little guy she's seen this year. By the time the team is ready to meet with you, you're frazzled too. You've done nothing but answer questions and watch your child be scrutinized for weeks. This tends to raise anxiety, perhaps expectations, and create a sense of unnecessary drama around the final wrap-up session. If you've been put through this, you know how frustrating it can be and how much doubt it can instill about the reliability of the diagnosis produced.

Now you know what a best-practice assessment looks like and what to seek for your child—or whether a diagnosis you've already received was based on reliable measures. The next chapter will tell you how to find this type of assessment, what it will entail, how you can prepare, and what you'll learn. If you've been through the process before, it will help you confirm that you've done enough and should get started on treatment or show you what to look for in a second opinion.

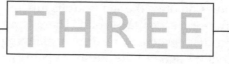

THREE

Setting a Course

NAVIGATING THE DIAGNOSTIC PROCESS
TO EMERGE WITH A PLAN

You might consider the preceding chapter your introduction to diagnostic theory. Now you're going to get into the practical aspect of diagnosis. How do you find a place to have your child assessed? Which types of experts will you meet, and what will they do during the evaluation? How can you prepare to play your role optimally? When the assessment is done, what will you get out of it—and how do you know if it's enough?

You may be more interested in that last question than the others if you're already involved in having your child evaluated. Remember, the goal is to emerge from the process with enough information to devise a plan aimed specifically at addressing your child's individual set of needs. It may be helpful to review the process to find out now whether any steps seem to have been skipped. When you're still working with these clinicians, it's easier to go back to them with additional questions than it might be months down the road. You can also take any questions that arise as you read this chapter to the feedback session, where you will hear the conclusions drawn from the findings of the evaluation. If you still don't feel entirely satisfied by the assessment process or conclusions, the last part of this chapter explains the value of second opinions.

Finding the Right Place for an Assessment

As I said in Chapter 2, if your child has screened positive for autism, there is no reason not to go straight to an autism specialty clinic if there is one in your area. The more urban the area in which you live, the better your chances of finding one. These clinics are really subspecialty clinics and most often are part of a child development center at a large community hospital, a department of child psychiatry at a medical school, or part of a clinical psychology or developmental/behavioral pediatrics training program.

The reason not to go straight to an autism specialty clinic, even if one is available to you, would be that it's clear your child has other specific difficulties such as significant motor delays, a seizure disorder, or a suspected diagnosis of a comorbid (at the same time) genetic disorder that will involve its own workup and treatment plans.

The other big factor in deciding where to seek diagnostic assessment is third-party insurance. In an attempt to contain costs, most insurance carriers try to limit coverage to fairly generic, superficial services where as much as possible can be "turfed" from them to some other fiduciary entity—like the schools. It's possible this is changing, but I wouldn't hold my breath. Parents who advocate strongly, call their insurance companies frequently, know exactly which billing (or CPT) codes will be covered, know which can be billed in conjunction with one another, and check in with the billing office of the assessment center before they go *may* feel less stressed by the time the day of the assessment rolls around. But insurance companies change rules and contracts with preferred providers faster than most twenty-year-old Hollywood starlets change boyfriends. Don't expect this part to be easy. If there are any choices to be made, and there is an autism clinic with a good reputation for individualized treatment planning, go with it. In the long run, you will learn more and take less grief than if you have a more superficial assessment and then find you need another because you're still not sure what to do next. You may have already learned this the hard way.

In fact many parents do. Some parents I meet have had many stops along the road before arriving on my doorstep, at an autism specialty clinic. All along, parents have been aware that there is a suspicion of autism, but the child has been sent off to the various "blind men" who have felt the bit of the elephant placed within their reach. This isn't bad. It can be like getting a second opinion about parts of the difficulty before you have a first (whole) opinion. As long as you eventually get that whole opinion, you should get the answers you need. But my preference will always be to send children straight from primary care to an autism clinic if that is the main suspected diagnosis because it is emotionally and economically less stressful on families who already are looking at a good-sized burden of care.

"Snowballing"

How do you know if you've found the right place to start having your child assessed? In market research there's a concept called "snowballing" that you can tap. It involves calling different people for their suggestions and then calling the people you've been told to call, till most everything seems to point in one direction. That's the person or team you see. You can start by calling friends who are connected to education, mental health services, or developmental services. You may end up talking to some really great professionals who you feel you connect with—but who tell you autism is not really their thing. Ask that person who to talk to next. My guess is that you will know when you have identified the right place to go.

The Different Kinds of Professionals Involved in Autism Assessment

Who will you meet as you and your child go through an autism assessment? What kinds of information will you be asked to provide? How stressful will this be for your child? This section reviews the ways you and your child can expect to be prodded and prompted to construct the picture needed to make a diagnosis and a treatment plan.

The Developmental or Clinical Psychologist

The psychologist you see should be a child specialist. In addition, it should be someone who specializes in assessment, not someone who is primarily a therapist. Family members or friends may recommend someone who for them has been the most wonderful psychologist in the world—but make sure autism is part of their world. Someone who is great at assessing school phobias or attention deficit disorder (ADD) may not have the specialized set of skills to assess for autism. The psychologist is often the "primary clinician" on a team in a specialty clinic. This means he will be the one to ask about your overall concerns, identify your goals for the assessment, take a history, usually coordinate the efforts of the rest of the team, and help select what specific assessment tools to use. In locales where there is no autism specialty clinic or team, it is certainly possible for a psychologist knowledgeable about autism to carry out the full assessment himself.

Another role, usually reserved for psychologists, is that of psychological testing (sometimes called "psych testing"), which can include cognitive testing (a term that basically means intelligence testing) or psychoeducational testing (which usually means how aspects of intelligence and ability define the child's capacities to function in an educational setting). Chapter 9 decribes for you how psychoeducational testing can be used to formulate IEP (individualized education program) goals. For now it's enough to be sure you know that this is a valuable part of assessment at any stage because it gives an overall review of the child's capacities, highlights relative strengths and weaknesses, and gives some way of predicting future development in children of school age or older. On the other hand, if a child does not yet have any "instructional control," meaning she has not yet had the opportunity to learn the "do something for me, and I'll give something to you" rule, the examiner need not have the materials from an overpriced IQ test tossed around the room to ascertain this. However, if there is any chance of learning about relative strengths and weaknesses, psychological testing should be included in an assessment.

MD Specialists: Child Psychiatrists, Developmental/Behavioral Pediatricians

Similarly, a child psychiatrist or developmental or behavioral pediatrician may be the primary clinician for a team assessment. These clinicians are usually not trained to use the full range of standard tests for assessing autism that a psychologist is more likely to be familiar with, but may bring other advantages. As MDs, they are better able to discuss and if necessary prescribe a psychoactive medicine as part of your child's treatment. Child psychiatrists tend to be best trained on the medication front, and developmental or behavioral pediatricians are also really helpful if genetic, metabolic, or neurological workups may also be called for as part of the comprehensive diagnostic assessment. One limitation to MDs as sole diagnostician/treatment planners is that few, with a couple of notable exceptions, have in-depth experience with the range of school programs for children with autism or with principles of applied behavior analysis—the main autism treatments.

Educational Specialists

Increasingly, as schools create autism-specific classrooms and other services, their intake and assessment teams may contain a core of evaluators (such as school psychologists, speech pathologists, classroom special education teachers) who have sought out additional training in autism, particularly expertise in using autism-specific standardized assessment tools. Such a specialty team may provide assessments that are particularly strong on very good treatment ideas. Diagnosis is not part of the specific training of either school psychologists or speech therapists, but much of the time this is not the most prominent goal of the assessment anyway, especially in a school-age child where diagnosis was clearly ascertained years ago. As part of a multidisciplinary or transdisciplinary team, the education professional is key to helping the rest of the team work with available resources, identify special areas of training that school staff may need to implement a treatment plan, or serve as a "translator" between medical and educational agencies.

Educational specialists usually test a child within their area of specialty. This can include psychoeducational testing carried out by school psychologists (who are usually, though not always, MA-level psychologists), language testing by a speech and language pathologist (more about this in the next section), or tests of motor and sensory function typically administered by an occupational or physical therapist.

Speech and Language Pathologists

Speech and language pathologists (sometimes referred to as SLPs) are trained to work with both speech *and* language problems: A child is said to have "language" problems when she's having difficulty learning what words mean (semantics), how to form phrases and sentences (grammar), and when and how to speak (language pragmatics). A child is said to have "speech" problems when she makes articulation errors (speaking indistinctly or mixing sounds up) or when she has more severe speech clarity issues like oral–motor apraxia or dyspraxia—meaning that the connection between the brain and the output devices (jaw, lips, tongue, voice) seems rather faulty. Most children with autism, though, suffer mainly from more basic *language* problems that affect comprehension and expression and less often from speech problems. Children with high-functioning autism and Asperger syndrome more often have mainly "language pragmatic" problems (for example, with taking turns in a conversation, maintaining a topic, and getting a conversation going). Some SLPs specialize in the language pragmatics problems of children on the autistic spectrum. These SLPs might run social skills groups where children receive supervised practice in listening to others, making conversation, and staying on the topic. The concerns the SLPs observe and characterize cut across many symptoms of autism since communication in general, and language in particular, is so closely tied to being social. A major area in the differential diagnosis of autism is severe language impairments of different types. (The term *differential diagnosis* essentially means "figuring out what else it could be.") This makes an SLP a critical part of any diagnostic team. On her own, she will be able to assess language difficulties of the types that children with autism experience, as well as devise treatment plans to address them. However, on her own, an SLP may or may not be in a position to diagnose autism. Many are excellent at differential diagnosis, but it depends on experience. Certainly an SLP is in a good position to know when to refer a child for an autism assessment.

Most often, SLPs test either receptive language (what a child can understand), expressive language (what a child can say), or a combination of the two, which can be helpful in contrasting the child's relative strengths and weaknesses communicatively. Common tests that a speech and language pathologist will give a child just learning to understand and talk include the PLS (Preschool Language Scale), the PPVT (Peabody Picture Vocabulary Test), and the EOWVT (Expressive One-Word Vocabulary Test). As language abilities include communicating in phrases and sentences, the verbal portion of intelligence tests can tell quite a bit of the story about a child's language strengths and weaknesses. There are also tests sometimes used specifically for language pragmatics that focus on the nonverbal part of communication—which not only includes staying on topic and making conversation, as mentioned earlier, but also assessing the way body language serves as an additional "grammar." This is important if we are to help a child develop overall communication skill competence. Typically developing young children actually master "talking" with body language (like gazing, pointing, and reaching) before they develop any oral speech.

Occupational Therapists

Many children with autism have difficulties taking in or making sense of different information that comes from the senses: Some children with autism cover their ears to certain sounds. Some children with autism seem deaf—but hearing tests show they aren't. There can also be olfactory problems: Some children smell everything; others put all sorts of things in their mouths indiscriminately. Some children with autism appear insensitive to pain, while others can't tolerate that tag at the back of a T-shirt. Some autistic children love to swing and bounce and can seem calmed by it, while others are much more cautious and fearful of new movement sensations. Overall, a fair number of children with autism have difficulty modulating responses to one or more kinds of these sensory stimuli. As a result, many occupational therapists who work with children with autism work on what is considered "sensory integration"—achieving better-modulated responses to these different kinds of sensations.

The jury is definitely still out on whether becoming desensitized to certain kinds of strong sensory inputs helps anything but the future likelihood of becoming overloaded by the same strong sensory inputs. However, some occupational therapists claim that less sensory over-response represents better sensory integration, which in turn may lead to being less symptomatic overall. The idea that sensory integration of some sort is achieved in any neurologically measurable way remains unproven. Therefore the value of desensitization activities like brushing a child with soft brushes, or having the child wear weighted vests or sit on bumpy cushions at school—all things that some occupational therapists recommend in the name of sensory integration—is questionable for most children with autism. Occupational therapists are usually part of a team autism assessment only when the assessment takes place at a center that provides assessment for a number of childhood difficulties. While it can be helpful to have an occupational therapist as part of an assessment team, addressing these sensory processing over- and underresponses is never as big a problem as helping the child develop social skills or learn to use words to communicate. While some autistic children like the activities designed to recalibrate sensory responses—like back rubs, weighted vests, deep pressure, or joint compression, there's no proof they are therapeutic on their own. A back rub can be seen as a reinforcer if a child likes it. What occupational therapy work can add to the autistic child's life may be really salient reinforcers (like back rubs) that can motivate the child in all sorts of learning situations. However, in isolation this "sensory integration" type of work an occupational therapist may do with a child with autism is likely not as valuable on its own as work on specific fine and gross motor delays—which should certainly also be assessed as part of a team assessment of any child with autism. Virtually always, you will be more concerned with helping your child develop social and language skills. That brings us to our next topic.

You, the Parents!

Who else is on the assessment team? You, of course. There is no team unless parents are on board. Parents are the key ingredient of any treatment plan. You work with everyone else to select the needed assessors, treatment planners, and treatment implementers. I know it doesn't always feel that way. It sure is possible to quietly abdicate this role and indicate to others that you are willing to be less rather than more active on your child's behalf. But he is yours and always will be. You are the one to whom all this will matter most in the end.

How do you assure your place on the team? Ask questions from the first moment you call anyone for an appointment. We have some parents who call us and simply leave a message saying "I'm calling because my baby's doctor, Dr. V, said I should, so I am calling to make an appointment." How does that sound to us? Like this parent cares deeply about what we'll do? Unfortunately not. We call back. We set up an appointment. But in the process we will try to show her what her role will be and the kinds of things she can ask us—and that we can answer. The next section explains how you can set things up to be proactive and seen from the get-go as your child's advocate.

Be Prepared!

When you meet with someone assessing your child, be prepared. This conveys your desire to be involved. If you've prepared well, you'll get much more out of the assessment. What will you need to do to prepare? First you will need to learn exactly who you will see, for how long, what you should bring, and how much time you will have to meet with the main clinician. If you are to meet with a medical resident or psychology intern, will you also see his or her supervisor? When and for how long? Can you request a particular doctor at the clinic if one has been recommended to you? (Don't assume you are going to see the head of the clinic if you go to a university hospital or to any big medical center.) If you're going to talk about educational issues, is the main clinician you will see conversant in all the educational and behavioral treatment models you want to discuss? (Not all MDs are.) If you are going to want to learn about medicines or biomedical approaches, is the main clinician you're going to see an MD—or especially knowledgeable about medical treatments for autism? (Not all PhDs are.) The soonest appointment may not be with the clinician who is most in demand, but rather some of his or her trainees. This is okay if you'll see the doctor you want for some of the time—because it will be part of the trainee's job to meet with his or her supervisor and fill the supervisor in on what's been learned. The time to ask who you will see is when you set up your appointment to have your child assessed; ask what the person's position is in the clinic and whether he or she is an MD, a PhD, or another specialist.

What to Take to an Assessment

When you set up an appointment for an assessment, always ask what you should bring. Records of your child's previous assessments, if any, will be helpful. Taking them to the appointment not only provides another "method" for the assessor to use to evaluate data on your child but also shows you are organized. You can ask ahead of time, but generally things like birth records and well-baby pediatric care records are not going to be reviewed as part of an autism assessment. If there were pregnancy or birth events you are concerned may be part of the reason your child has his difficulties, though, include those records. The records that can be most helpful are earlier diagnostic assessments, speech and language assessments, and school or Early Start intakes, as these can be used to benchmark a child's developmental progress from each earlier age at which the child was seen.

If you haven't done so already, this is a perfect time to start a binder of all this information about your child. Use dividers to separate medical records from ones from a speech therapist, teachers, psychologists, and so on. If you have an initial assessment from someone followed by progress reports, put the initial assessment first, followed by the progress reports in chronological order. Ask ahead of time if you should bring in photocopies you can give the assessment team for its chart. It will be easier on you to just hand over copies of everything than to be flipping pages of a binder during an assessment when you should be listening or answering questions. If you have copies with you, you can hand them over to the clinician and then refer to your copy, still in its place in your binder. Ask if you should make copies of IEPs or IFSPs (individualized family service plans) or IPPs (individualized program plans)—the plans that various agencies give you for your child. While these can be helpful for other professionals to review, they are not infrequently printed on colored paper—and photocopy really poorly unless you are careful.

Some families I see do go overboard with this preparing. They put the records they are bringing *me* in a binder. This is awkward, because the doctor is most likely going to be adding them to a medical chart that is organized the way all his other charts are—so he can find things again. Mailing them ahead of time can be helpful and considerate, but ask first. If you don't send it to the exact right address at a major medical center, it could end up anywhere but with the rest of the information on your child. Faxing, Express Mailing, and so on, are usually over the top unless they've been requested for a special reason—like your taking a last-minute cancellation appointment. These days there are draconian rules around patient confidentiality—so e-mailing records may cause more trouble for the recipient than it's worth.

Before you go to an assessment is a perfect time to make a list of the specific questions you want to have answered. You might jot your questions under these headings (in addition to others that come to mind):

- Diagnosis
- Level of Cognitive Functioning
- Language Abilities
- Best Way to Teach
- Best Way to Motivate
- Proposed Treatment Setting(s)
- The Future

If you plan to hand a list of questions to the clinician in charge (a very good idea), keep your questions succinct so the clinician will have time to read them (and be sure to answer them) before the end of the feed-back session. If you're having assessment and feedback in one session, give the questions at the beginning so your discussions will encompass the things you want to learn more about. Remember, this session is happening to help you and your child. The more help you ask for, the more you will get.

Who Should Be There?

Take Support Along

If a child is going for a first diagnostic assessment, it is *really* impor-tant for both parents to be there, especially if this is the day you're going to learn whether your child has autism. That is news that is going to affect both of you. It is certainly true that each parent can be expected to react differently, and we will discuss this in detail in Chapter 4, when we talk about the effect autism can have on a fam-ily. For now, suffice it to say, if at all possible, it would be good for both parents to be there if both are involved in the child's upbring-ing. For parents who are alone, or parents who have a spouse that simply can't be there, consider taking along a friend or other family member. Getting the diagnosis is not good news, and no one should be alone for this.

On a more practical level, I know that it can be really hard to hear anything after you've heard the diagnosis. Someone else who is not quite so close to the situation, such as a grandparent, aunt, or uncle, can do this listening for you. Take a tape recorder too. (Ask about a tape recorder in advance, however, since not all clinicians are comfort-able with this.) The purpose of taping a feedback session is to allow you to feel it is okay not to "hear" what is being said at the moment. You can listen to it again later. When you listen later, you may be in a better state of mind to make a list of questions you can make sure are answered in the clinicians' report of the assessment, by e-mail, or over the phone.

Take a Teacher Along

If you're going for an assessment of a school-age child, it can be very helpful to take along a teacher, therapist, or other person involved in the child's treatment, even his one-to-one paraprofessional aide. Hav-

ing this person there will allow the clinicians to get some direct information about how the child is doing in treatment. If appropriate,
clinicians may even want to see the person involved in the child's
treatment doing a little work with him. That makes a great, concrete
basis for discussing any new ideas or modifications to current activities. Sometimes a child acts rather different for a teacher or therapist
than for a parent. If one has better instructional control than the other,
it can be much easier for the clinician to point out what seems to be
working and what is not and what seems to be effective, rather than
putting a parent in the difficult position of having to tell treating professionals why she likes one of them better than the other. If you do
take a professional with you, ask ahead of time when it will be most
helpful to have that person along and plan how long that person can or
should stay. Make sure the team doing the assessment understands
this from the outset so it can be incorporated into their scheduling during the assessment.

The Case Conference:
The Part Parents Seldom See

The day of your assessment has come. Various people have run in and
out of the examining room. Your child is seen by several people. You
are taken here and there. You are asked lots of questions, fill in or hand
in all kinds of forms. Then you are told the assessment is done. You are
to come back next week, next month, or after lunch to learn what has
been concluded. How are the conclusions you will be hearing about
reached?

Assuming you have had a team assessment of some sort, the various evaluators will need an opportunity to talk with one another.
(Even an individual evaluator will likely need time to score tests and
questionnaires and perhaps give a phone call to teachers or other assessors who already know the child.) In a good-quality assessment the
team should meet together so that everyone can share their impressions and observations. This is the core of the multitrait/multimethod
philosophy that was described in Chapter 2. Everybody's impressions
and measures need to get lined up so a comprehensive view of the
child can be passed on to you.

My own feeling is that it's best if the case conference results are
conveyed to parents by one or two of the people with whom the par-

ents have spent the most time. I like sitting around a play room rather than meeting over a big official-looking conference table. What can be very hard on parents is you against a whole table of professionals who are going to take turns telling you "what is." It's this setup that makes most parents I know begin to feel that advocating for their child is an "us against them" proposition.

Different agencies have different policies, but you can ask if it would be possible to meet in a way that isn't going to make you more nervous than you already are. For example, after a school-based assessment you may get many different reports. If you read them ahead of time, it may not be necessary to have the occupational therapist, adaptive PE teacher, inclusion specialist, *and* resource teacher at your three-year-old's first IEP. Sometimes a school will ask all these people to be present just to show you that everyone cares. However, having two or three people who sit there and say little or nothing doesn't help you. These folks would probably rather be off actually working with children anyway.

The Feedback Session: What You Need to Learn at the Parent Debriefing Session

Remember that list I suggested you make before going into an assessment? It forms the basis of the topics you can expect to cover in a diagnostic feedback session or a treatment planning session. Let's go through each topic in more depth. These are the kinds of questions you should have answers to by the time you leave a diagnostic and/or treatment planning evaluation. If for any reason you don't get through your list, it will be important to schedule another visit soon or to finish up on the phone or by e-mail. In my clinic, we have a follow-up coordinator whom parents are encouraged to call with any questions that come up on that drive home—or anytime after the visit. Given that option, about a quarter of our parents do call. Sometimes they just want a phone number for an agency or provider we've mentioned, or the name of a book we've recommended. But sometimes a very stressed-out parent didn't "hear" the diagnosis; or Mom and Dad heard different diagnoses. If that happens to you, it's completely understandable, because the assessment can be such a stressful thing. If you need more information, don't fight about what was meant by what was said—just leave your assessment with a name and number you can call to get that follow-up support.

Diagnosis

If we're talking about an initial assessment or a diagnostic "second" (or third) opinion, you should hear about your child's diagnosis. It should be framed in terms of the diagnostic criteria promulgated by the American Psychiatric Association in the DSM-IV-TR (the text revision of the fourth edition of the *Diagnostic and Statistical Manual of Mental Disorders*). The twelve specific areas of possible difficulty are listed on page 60.* There may not be time to go through each one, but maybe there will be. You should at least come away knowing which of these twelve criteria were concerns about your child and what you may have described or the doctor may have observed that was considered a problem.

Then you need to understand the specific diagnosis: What's the verdict? Autism? PDD? (Do you really understand the difference between the two? If not, this will be the time to ask.) If it's autism, why isn't it PDD? If it's PDD, why isn't it autism? If you have questions about Asperger syndrome or if someone else has suggested this to you, *do* ask. Does the doctor think this diagnosis is likely to change? How often does the doctor see a child like yours getting a "downgraded" diagnosis (moving from "autism" to "PDD" or "PDD" to "Asperger")? Many parents do ask if their child will get worse. Don't worry about that. If she gets proper treatment, she won't. But it might feel good to ask that and hear the answer nevertheless.

Level of Cognitive Functioning and Language Abilities

Where does mental development fit in? Overall, is your child seen as functioning the same as or below others his age? With respect to understanding language? With respect to using language? When will he start talking? Will he start talking? Do some autistic kids never talk? Do you think he could be one of them? As far as nonlanguage intelligence goes, is he doing better? (Most children with autism are.) Does it seem like the child has mental retardation? What is this based on? Was the cognitive or language testing done as part of this assessment considered valid, or were there too many problems with behavior, cooperation, and motivation to say for sure? Will he be likely to function in the mentally retarded range when he's older? Does the doctor think

---

*American Psychiatric Association. (2000). *Diagnostic and statistical manual of mental disorders* (4th ed., text rev.). Washington, DC: Author.

The Twelve Diagnostic Criteria
for the DSM-IV-TR Autism Spectrum Disorders

Given the child's developmental level, which of these is atypical?

A. Atypical social interactions	
1	Impaired nonverbal behaviors such as eye contact, facial expressions, body posture, and gestures used in social interaction
2	Lack of peer relationships
3	Doesn't try to share enjoyment, interests, or achievements with others, such as by leading others to, pointing to, or showing off things of interest
4	Failure to demonstrate social-emotional reciprocity
B. Atypical communication	
1	Delayed in spoken language without compensating through other means of communication
2	Noticeable inability to start or sustain conversation
3	Stereotyped repetitive or idiosyncratic use of language, as in echolalia
4	Doesn't engage in varied, spontaneous, make-believe play or social imitation
C. Atypical responses to social and perceptual stimuli in the environment	
1	Preoccupied by abnormally intense or focused stereotyped or restrictive patterns of interest
2	Adheres compulsively to nonfunctional rituals or routines
3	Stereotyped and repetitive movements
4	Persistent preoccupation with parts of objects, such as their sensory aspects

How many and which criteria must be met to get a diagnosis?

Autism	At least two from A, at least one each from B and C, and six overall; onset before two years old
PDDNOS	At least one from A, one from B, with or without any from C; onset before two years old
Asperger syndrome	At least one from A, one from C, with or without any from B, and single words by age two and phrases by three

treatment will make him less behind? In what ways? These are important things for you to learn about because the child's overall rate of development is going to be your meter for how much change you can expect in a year's time—and how far ahead of the present levels of performance those IEP goals should be set.

Best Way to Teach: Learning Styles

"What has been learned about my child's learning style? Is she a visual learner? If so, do you think she will be helped by picture schedules, picture communication, or visual schedules?"

"Why is she so repetitive? Should I let her repeat or do the same things over and over? Does she 'need' to do it? What can go wrong if we try to make her stop?"

"She has so many routines; is that bad for her? I think routines help her know what to expect; do they? Should I stop them then?"

"She likes the computer so much; is that good for or bad for her? What about TV?"

"What is she paying attention to? Is she really understanding everything and just choosing to ignore us?"

The things that have been learned by those doing your child's assessment should give you a start at understanding the answers to these questions. In Chapter 6, I'll show you how you can delve more deeply into the answers to these questions yourself—which will guide you in understanding these learning styles for yourself. As your child gains new skills, you are the one who will need to be alert to how her learning is changing—to get new assessments and new treatment plans.

What's the Best Way to Motivate and to Deal with Behavioral Problems?

"He's not toilet trained. Should I be working on that now? I've tried to train him the same way as his brother and it doesn't work; what should I do now?"

"He doesn't eat anything. He eats everything. He eats only crunchy things. Why? Can I change that?"

"He doesn't listen; he's not safe when we go out in public. I can't leave him home all the time; what should I do?"

"He doesn't care if he's punished. He *likes* getting a time-out; so

how can I make him stop hurting the baby when she cries, . . .
running out the front door, . . . pulling what he wants out of
the fridge?"

What Kind of Teaching Setting?

"Everyone says she should get an ABA (applied behavior analysis) program. What does that actually mean?"

"From what I understand of ABA programs, I'm not sure she does
need it."

"What are my other choices? What about going to school?"

"Should she be in a special ed class or included with the other kids
of the same age?"

"What's good about special ed?"

"What's good about inclusion?"

"What does it mean that the school wants to mainstream her? Will
she get enough help that way?"

"The school said I could have a one-to-one aide if you said she
needed it. How come you think she does (doesn't) need one?"

"What's a TEACCH class? I was told my district does TEACCH
for autism."

"Is what the school is going to offer us enough? Does my child
need forty hours a week? Which hours do I count?"

"Do I need to get my own speech and language pathologist? Occupational therapist?"

"What about after school? What kinds of activities are good for
him then? Should he go (not go) to day care? Do I need a one-
to-one at home after school? On the weekends?"

"What's my role in all of this?"

The Séance: What Does the Future Hold?

"Doctor, I know you don't have a crystal ball, but . . . "

"When will my child learn to talk? Understand me?"

"Will she still have this when she grows up? How can we know
what to plan for? Does this mean I should stop putting money
in her college fund? Will she get married someday? Have a
job? Drive a car? Live independently?"

"How will we be able to tell if we're doing the right things for her?
Making the right choices? How can we tell if she is fulfilling
her potential?"

How Much Assessment Is Enough?

How will you know when you have had your child fully assessed? This question can be answered in many different ways. First, if every one of the questions above that apply to your child has been answered to your satisfaction for the present time, you've had enough assessment for now. It's time to get to work. But maybe only some of your questions have been answered. Maybe you've been told there is no answer to most of these questions. If you still want more answers before you feel you can act, get more assessment.

It's an individual thing. The purpose of initial diagnostic assessments is to qualify a child for services and to specify what those initial services should be. If you don't like what you've been told, or if it doesn't resonate with you as true, it's going to be hard to get behind the recommendations that have been made. If the recommendations have lacked specificity (like take him to the schools for special education and get speech therapy), you may need more assessment. Which approaches should the speech therapist consider? Which approaches does the assessor think will work best and why? Does this make sense to you?

The bottom line is that you can always seek more assessment. Have you gotten to the point where you feel you know enough to start looking for treatment? Plunging into treatment is scary. Getting more assessment can put that moment on hold. The trade-off is how much more you really need to learn versus how much can be gained from getting started with some available resources. As you learn more, you can always tailor or change what you are doing. It can be hard to judge whether a test that has not yet been done is really necessary or if testing that has already been done gives essentially the same information. If you ask what a proposed test will tell in terms of informing possible treatments, you'll be in a better position to know whether that test will offer you anything over what you already have.

Do Schools Do Fair Assessments?

Some parents are concerned about the validity of tests done by schools. You may be concerned that the main outcome of the school's testing was to exclude your child from some service or another. Some parents worry that their child will be judged less able and then be less fully served because he behaved badly and, as a result, did poorly on the school's testing.

These are understandable concerns. You might consider addressing them by asking if you can be there to observe the testing. But some
assessors don't want the parent in the room because it changes the information they can get about how ready your child is for different
kinds of teaching (like following instructions that are only verbal,
needing frequent breaks, and so on). Fair enough. However, many
schools have a room with an observation window or partition where
you can watch without being noticed. Alternatively, the tester may be
willing to videotape all or part of an assessment session so you can
later see whether your child was doing what he could do. Most standardized tests, used properly, don't leave much "wiggle room" for
bias, so this is usually not a big worry. However, having someone unfamiliar and unattuned test your child, or testing him in an environment
with lots of competing stimulation, like a classroom, may not be sam-
pling your child at his best or even at his "typical." Conversely, certain
tests are subject to memory effects, and the child's performance may
reflect what he has learned from the last administration rather than being a pure measure of ability. Giving a test too many times so that there
is a memory effect may mask the true difficulties that need to be
treated. (For example, your child might have difficulty with more than
memorization.) Because of this, there are rules about how often certain
tests, particularly IQ tests, can be repeated. So, if a test isn't done, there
may be a reason that can be explained to you.

The Three E's:
Expertise, Experience, and Evangelical Fervor

Who do you trust if you get different assessments and it seems like different people are saying different things? I put my money on expertise.
How long has this assessor/treatment recommender been working
with children with autism? The longer the person has been in the picture, the better idea he or she will have of the "bigger picture" and not
just the treatment du jour. Someone who is very knowledgeable about
low-functioning children with autism may be at a loss in making recommendations for high-functioning children and vice versa. Some
people concentrate on early intervention, others on the life skills for
older children. Ask what an assessor has the greatest experience at.
Rely on an assessor who knows about what you need to learn about.
Beware of people who speak of their recommendations with evangeli-
cal fervor. A big problem today is "assessments" by evaluators at private agencies who have a service to sell. About 100% of the time, it

turns out that your child *does* need the service they happen to sell. Now it is certainly fair, best practice even, for any service provider to carry out some assessment before starting treatment to learn where to start, as well as to get baseline data to compare to later progress reports. However, using assessment as a marketing tool on parents of children with autism who are desperate to get started—and get started any way they can—is just not quite fair. If the assessor is also a treatment provider, ask what other treatments that provider knows how to use. If the answer is that the recommended treatment is the only one he or she knows, you may well want to consider further assessment for treatment recommendations from someone experienced in a variety of techniques.

Learning the Lingo: "Are These Folks Really Saying the Same Thing?"

The more you talk to different professionals, the more you will hear different ways of saying the same thing. We have already talked about the blind-men-feeling-the-elephant conundrum; this is a variation. If you don't understand, ask. For example, I have parents who tell me that they have been told their child does not have autism but has a multisystem developmental disorder (MSDD). Okay . . . well, as it happens, *autism* and *autistic disorder* are terms from the standards of the American Psychiatric Association's DSM and the World Health Organization's ICD (International Classification of Diseases), which are what 90–95% of clinicians use. However, in the United States, the National Center for Clinical Infant Programs (a professional organization for those dealing with children under three years old) has laid out its own set of diagnostic criteria for very young children. MSDD is in there. Many of these children have PDDNOS; many more have autism—and they do also meet criteria for MSDD. It's not like they have one and not the other. Same thing with some cases of an expressive language disorder and dyspraxia—it means you can't talk well (and it means you're talking to either a school psychologist, who said "expressive language disorder," or to a neurologist, who said "dyspraxia").

There are other terms that are bandied about with little to help you pin down exact meaning: The two big ones that come to mind are *early* and *intensive*. How early is early? When is it not early anymore? Early intervention really means getting started as soon as you can. Some parents hear about the "window of opportunity" of which early intervention takes advantage. We are not talking triple-paned, double-hung here. The "window" is not going to slam shut on your child's third birthday, insulating him from any further learning. Also, intervention is not just formal services, but in large part, as we will discuss in Chapter 4, what parents themselves provide their child in the way of a rich, comprehensible environment in which he can navigate with increasing independence. So even implementation of good parent training via reading, training workshops, home visitors, and so on marks the "earliest" interventions for most children.

What about intensive? If one more parent tells me that he read on the Web that his child needs forty hours a week of one-to-one, I will scream into my hand. The truth is, we don't fully understand what the components of "intensive" are. Obviously, the more time the child is in treatment, the more treatment he gets. However, what the active ingredients of "treatment" are remains obscure. Is it the amount of time the child is being asked to pay attention to an instruction or a demonstration? Is it the amount of time he is actually attending? Is it the amount of time he is working to solve a problem or follow an instruction? Is it the amount of time he provides accurate response that reinforces what is being taught? Another dimension has to do with what the child is being taught. If the child is being asked to do things for which he has prerequisite skills, fine. But what about things (like in an inclusion setting) that may still be above his skill level? All parents realize that their children "connect" with some teachers and therapists better than others. Should we assign "bonus" hours to work done with the talented teachers and discount the hours spent with new therapists who muck around, unsure of how to engage the child?

I like to respond to the "forty hours" question with a bit of a jolting response, which I hope will get parents thinking about the substantive issues here. I'll say, "No, forty hours is not enough; your child needs intervention twenty-four hours a day, seven days a week." At first this seems frightening, not to mention impossible. But really, 24/7 intervention is what parenting is all about. With a child with autism you surely need added expertise and more respite, but meaningfully structuring all the child's experiences leverages the potential that any moment will become a "teaching" moment.

What a "Second Opinion" Can and Can't Do

There are many times when I will be lecturing at a conference on autism, and a parent will come up to me at the break and say, "We already have our diagnosis, but we're not sure if we should be doing X or Y—that's why we came today. Really, which do you think we should be doing?" My answer is always that it depends on your child. I ask about the diagnostic assessment the child did have and what treatments were recommended based on what was learned at that time about the child's learning styles. In response, I am not infrequently told that the diagnosis was just that, a diagnosis—followed by a suggestion to go to the school and get services.

If this is what has happened to you, you are likely in need of a "second opinion." This is not to suggest that a diagnosis without a treatment plan is wrong, but that you have gotten only half the story. I would suspect that if all you got from a diagnostic assessment was a diagnosis (and no treatment plan), going back to the same folks won't be the best move.

The best thing about a second opinion is that it can tell you what you've already been told. It makes the diagnosis more real. It can help galvanize the resolve you need to get started on a treatment plan. If you go into a second opinion visit understanding that different clinicians are likely to say things in a slightly different way, you'll be prepared. Remember that the substance should be the same—and if not, you are there to find out why opinions differ. Sometimes opinions about diagnosis or prognosis may come across differently at a different clinic. This should not be a big worry—as long as you feel confident that there is substantial agreement over what direction to take in treatment.

"Is It True Doctors Hate Patients Who Want a Second Opinion?"

Some parents don't mention when they come to me that they have already had an earlier diagnostic assessment. Others mention it only once they feel they have gotten to know me a bit. Still others state up front that they have had other assessments but haven't brought them because they know doctors all stick together and they want a fresh look at their child. Fine. It is your prerogative as a parent to proceed in a way that develops your confidence in the information you obtain. A good clinician should not be defensive about the fact that you consulted someone earlier and want to understand any differences in what each professional has recommended. A good clinician should not feel threatened if you say that next week you are also going to be seeing Dr. A or Dr. B, and you want to wait and see what that person has to say. Treatment recommendations should be logical and rationally defensible. Anyone who makes you feel like you should do as he or she says "because I said so" doesn't have a good enough reason for you not to question his or her directives.

Diagnosis Shopping and Doctor Hopping

Some parents shop for diagnoses. Some doctors will give parents the diagnosis they want, especially if it's felt that the diagnosis will allow access to services. I don't happen to do things that way. I call it like it is. To the extent that a diagnosis is of any use, its use, as was said earlier, is to be a shorthand for treatment needs. If a child needs some treatments designed for a child with autism but not others, he should have what he needs, not the parts he doesn't need. The important thing is that your child have his needs considered in the careful way that has been described so that the treatments recommended to you take advantage of unique strengths that can be recruited to help develop abilities that have, up till now, lagged behind. It can be harder work for the doctor to advocate for more specifically tailored services, but if that's what a patient needs, the doctor should say so in a way that explains and justifies why such services are needed.

"What If My Child's Not Autistic? Should I Keep Reading This Book?"

Some of you reading this book will have made it through one or more good diagnostic assessments and come to understand that what your child has is *not* an autism spectrum disorder. Or maybe you've been told your child has pervasive developmental disorder or that he may be developing Asperger syndrome—but that it is too early to tell for sure. Do you keep reading? Please do.

Autism is not a discrete have-it or not-have-it disease like cancer. It is a disorder, more like diabetes or asthma, which can be very severe and affect everything or just minor, requiring some greater consciousness about diet or an effort to stay away from allergens. In Chapter 6, we'll start talking about autism spectrum disorders as a series of autism-specific learning disabilities (ALDs). This gives us a way of breaking down all the symptoms associated with autism spectrum disorders and systematically addressing each that's an issue for a particular child. If your child was assessed to have *some* but not *enough* symptoms to meet the full criteria for autism, or maybe not enough symptoms to qualify as PDD, your child may still have some of these ALDs. If some of these barriers to learning are present for your child, he may indeed benefit from treatments designed to help these specific disabilities. Read on.

So Now You Know: What Next?

For families, the day of the diagnosis is the day of the "shot heard round the world." Everything changes, yet everything stays the same until you start to take action. In the next chapter we'll talk about mustering your resources, gathering your wits about you, and preparing to follow through on the plan that is beginning to take shape now that you know what's wrong.

PART II

Outfitting Yourself to Help Your Child

Your destination is the optimal treatment plan for your child. The "map" is the information provided by the diagnostic assessment. If you've just read Part I, you've either confirmed that the diagnostic process has already pointed you in the direction you need to go or determined that you need to turn back and get a better map.

If you're ready to go—onward! The next two chapters will help you pack for the journey. Your home, your family, the services you choose for your child, and the providers you select to implement them are all critical resources. The next two chapters are intended to help organize you—inside and out: On the home front, you need to take stock of what all this means to you as a person, to your marriage, and to any other children you may have. With your internal resources mustered, you'll then need to learn how others can best be of help to your family and your child, and who these others are.

You've undoubtedly read over and over that your child will need what amounts to full-time intervention. This is true in the sense that every waking moment of your child's life can and should be a learning opportunity. And because, realistically, you can't (and shouldn't want to) install a twenty-four-hour treatment team in your home, many of these opportunities can, with only moderate tweaking to normal family life, be created by you. Chapter 4 will show you how to do this, particularly in ways that will fit into your ordinary routine. Your child with autism can learn good behavior, routines, and even language from daily family goings-on just as any other child. Meanwhile, you need to learn to protect the irreplaceable resource of your family by maintaining some balance between what you do for the child with autism and how you meet everyone else's needs.

The other resources you need, obviously, are the services and providers that make up your child's treatment plan. The selection process, unfortunately, isn't as straightforward as you might hope. Autism has become a booming business, and there are plenty of snake oil salesmen out there as well as plenty of well-meaning people who just don't really understand autism. You need to become your own *Consumer Reports* investigative reporter as you consider different treatments that will become available, and Chapter 5 gives you tools for doing that.

FOUR

The Balanced
Family

"ADJUST YOUR OWN FACE MASK
BEFORE ATTEMPTING TO HELP OTHERS"

In Chapter 3, I said that a child with autism needs intervention twenty-four hours a day, seven days a week. In the broadest terms, treatment of autism is about providing constant, consistent, developmentally accessible learning experiences that cumulatively facilitate the child's ability to learn as the result of his own efforts. Clearly, a lot of that intervention is going to be up to you.

Most parents throw themselves heart and soul into this task. Unfortunately, many forget that, if they lose themselves, their child will become an emotional orphan. A child with autism is a child first, autistic second; he needs a life and a home as well as treatment. In this chapter, we're going to discuss how you and your family can accommodate your autistic child's needs, but also do a good job meeting everyone else's.

Naturally this balance will benefit your family collectively and individually. But it also falls right in line with working toward the best outcome for your child. Without a strong home base, you can't really focus your energies effectively on getting the help your child needs. As you'll read in the next chapter, just staying on top of treatment advances and ensuring that your child gets the best services from the best providers available to you is going to take a lot of time and effort. Add being a "provider" yourself and it's clear that you're going to need a strong family with the flexibility to roll with the needs of the autistic child without sapping your strength halfway through the labyrinth.

Doing the Best for Your Child at Home

That feeling of panic starts to set in: It's too late already. We should have known about this sooner. We should have listened to my mother/ your mother/our neighbor the former speech therapist/your sister-in-law's sister who has a child with autism. What if it *is* too late?

Every parent who has just heard the diagnosis of autism feels like he or she should have gotten started on getting help for the child yesterday. But your child's learning will occur over a lifetime, just as it does for any child. You have time. And the first thing you can do to contribute to your child's learning at home is to be a good model, by demonstrating caring, loving relationships, and provide a rich environment, where the child has many opportunities to experience new things. The child with autism will need special help to perceive and understand the same things as his siblings. His interests and activities will likely shape up differently. The child with autism does fit into his family differently. But his need for his family's love is the same. Accepting that the child with autism is the same as and different from siblings allows him acceptance and also acknowledges his special needs.

Next, you'll need to set up formal learning opportunities at home. Then I'll tell you how to avoid sacrificing your lives in the process, including being sure to count the informal learning opportunities that you naturally provide as part of your considerable accomplishments on your child's behalf.

Making Space for a Home Program

Many children with autism start with at least some home component to their treatment. The very intensive one-to-one services that so many children with autism need as part of initial treatment are mainly available on a home outreach basis. (Increasingly, however, schools are starting to offer one-to-one classrooms for the youngest children, and this can be a fine alternative.) One advantage of having a home program initially is that it's a great chance for you to get some ideas of how your child can learn and then to find ways to use those approaches yourself when tutors or therapists aren't around.

Having a "home program" usually means setting aside as your child's home teaching area a room or part of a room that isn't used for anything else during the day. Some families can devote an entire bedroom, lining the walls with bookcases and cubbies containing well-organized sets of teaching materials. I can think of two families who went a bit over the top, emptying out their living rooms of the usual living room contents, making a real classroom within the home. These living rooms virtually announced, "We don't live here anymore; life is only about our autistic son." In both cases, there were younger siblings, the houses were big enough to find space elsewhere, but it was clearly a lifestyle choice. The point is, your child's treatment will require allocation of special resources—like giving up a guest bedroom or moving the child's dresser into the hall to make room for a work table in his bedroom—but shouldn't become the literal center of family life. Many things need to take place in a family—like a happy marriage and well-cared-for siblings. Think about this too when you start to rearrange your house for treatment.

Depending on a child's learning needs, your home may need other modifications. For preverbal children, we set up a VIA (visual interaction augmentation) program (described in my book *Helping Children with Autism Learn*; see Resources at the end of this book), which means the house gets Velcroed in all the relevant places with photos of the things the child knows and loves best. Other things the child likes to get and use for herself (like DVDs or favorite snacks) are put out of reach so that a very motivating opportunity to communicate is created whenever the child happens to have a particular object she desires in mind.

Kill Your Television

Often parents think of what they need to do, but not what they need to avoid doing. For example, a home may need to be redesigned so that after hours of home-based treatment, with new information being given to the child every minute, opportunities for passive stimulation are limited. Take television, for example. When I watch home videos of children with autism in their own homes, I'm amazed at how many not only have a giant screen TV but have one playing when no one seems to be watching (and even when a videotape to show the doctor is being made). TV can be a meaningful and educational tool as part of the full scope of a child's education, but no household should have it on like background sound. Autistic children are generally already having a hard time discriminating what sounds to pay attention to, and there is some good evidence that these "noise" problems are at the core of their auditory processing difficulties.

So turn off the TV when no one is watching. Better yet, put it in a room that is not conducive to other activity and limit the time your autistic child—and, while you're at it, your other children—can watch. TV can be used as a reward for a child with autism. It can be used to encourage your child to model peers. It can be used to promote more imaginative play through encouragement of "playlalia"—in this case, imitating how kids on TV play. But if you need a babysitter, get a babysitter.

It's not just televisions that can be countertherapeutic. Any toy that encourages highly repetitive, unvaried play when the child is left on her own is not good. This includes so-called educational electronic toys and computers. Repetition is mental downtime compared to the learning that results from the varied exploration of typically developing children. This doesn't mean you have to put up all toys that, left to her own devices, your child will use repetitively. Instead it means that the pleasurable drive for repetition with the toy needs to be channeled into more productive learning opportunities through intervention so that productive learning becomes more pleasurable and intrinsically motivating.

Homes also need to be made autistic-child-proof. You probably already know this, but this is way more child-proof than child-proof. The child with autism is nothing if not an instrumental learner. If there is something he wants or somewhere he wants to go, he will figure it out using reasoning skills that leave you wondering why he can't match a red teddy bear to a red square. Not only does your house need to be safe; it needs to afford few opportunities for inappropriate behavior so you can focus on rewarding what your child does that is aimed at benefiting others, rather than always punishing what he's doing wrong.

"How Will I Know If My Child Is Getting Enough?"

Many families quickly set about getting services in place and within three to four months have a full complement of services up and running. Typically home-based programs start at 25% to 50% of full strength, going up to the planned number of hours within the first couple of months. Some children with home programs have them in the afternoon and go to school in the morning (or vice versa). Some children attend a special day class three to five mornings per week and attend a typical preschool on the other mornings or in the afternoons. All this depends on a plan tailored to your child's particular learning needs.

Parents often ask, "What hours do I count?" Forty hours seems to have acquired magical properties. (Is this because Americans work forty-hour weeks, so it seems a child should too?) The idea of forty hours came from the original Lovaas study on ABA/DTT (applied behavior analysis/discrete trial training; see more on this program in Chapters 7 and 8). What it really showed was that children whose hours were filled did better than those with more minimal intervention. In Lovaas's original work, parents were trained as "senior therapists," meaning "treatment" in some form really continued whenever parent and child interacted.

"Enough" intervention is when the child's hours are full. This means that if you have a younger child who still naps or needs a quiet time after lunch or later in the afternoon, that is a legitimate way to fill hours as well as with therapy. (You can't efficiently teach a child who wants to be asleep.) This means that so-called full-time intervention understandably involves fewer hours for a younger child than an older one. Children spend time being driven back and forth from school, Grandma's, play dates, and the speech therapist's office, and this fills the hours of the day as well. If you work nine to five for a salary, your employer doesn't deduct your lunch hour and bathroom breaks from your forty hours.

The point is that you shouldn't get too hung up on the number of hours. Instead, focus on how much of his time your child has opportunities for *meaningful engagement* with tutors and teachers as well as with you. How much of your child's time is spent doing things that keep her mentally challenged, not just in therapy activities but in other necessary activities of life? Most important is that the *content* of the intervention be developmentally appropriate and make the knowledge presented understandable to your child.

Fitting Yourself into Your Toddler's Busy Life

What's meaningful engagement? How many hours do you schedule for that? Is it an excuse for the school to give you fewer services? Am I implying that I expect *you*, the parent, who has no training in special education, to be responsible for teaching your child?

Yes. That's exactly what I mean. As the parent, you are not just the program manager or "general contractor" for your child's house of knowledge. You are also a builder. In fact, you are the guy who shows up with the cement truck. All the direct one-to-one teaching in the world will not find its way to becoming meaningful and functional, and thereby reinforcing for your child, if there are no opportunities to use emerging skills in a way that relates to making her world a place she can better understand and control. The everyday experiences that parents normally have with their children are the cement that bonds lessons learned in therapy to meaningful actions and activities.

One of the great strengths—and, if you're not careful, great limitations—of the autistic learner is that the child is always interested in learning about things that help him get what he wants or that gratify his interests. The child with autism tends to be much less interested in learning about things simply because they appear interesting to you or to others. One of the key contributions to our understanding of how children with autism learn comes from the work of those like Laura Schreibman and Bob and Lynn Koegel on what they call *pivotal responding*. They emphasize the need to create a press for the child with autism to get information to get something he wants. This is how you build a sense of intrinsic reinforcement in a child with autism.

Why is this so important? Many ABA/DTT or otherwise intensive one-to-one programs rely on external rewards like foods, preferred play opportunities, or tokens to earn these in the future. This works—but is very different from what reinforces the ongoing learning of the typically developing child. To move the child with autism closer to being able to learn from the same experiences that other children at the same developmental level do, parents need to create those presses. They need to take what is first being understood in a direct teaching format and find creative ways to make that knowledge work in the child's self-interest. If, for example, your child was learning the names of shapes and likes to see them drawn, you could use bath time to get her to name shapes and colors and then draw them together hand over hand on the wall of the tub.

This is meaningful engagement. This is where you fit very importantly into the life of your child with autism. There is, in fact, good reason to believe that these types of learning experiences are even more valuable than the ones embedded in drills logged in a data sheet that demonstrates "skill acquisition." Until your child can use her knowledge of colors and shapes to make interesting things happen in the part of her world that is experienced daily, she has not really mastered or acquired anything—as a data sheet might suggest.

At-Home Learning for Your School-Age Child

Pretty much the same thing goes for school-age children. If your child leaves for school at 8:00 and gets home at 3:00, scheduling another two hours of one-to-one tutoring denies him the opportunity to practice the knowledge acquired at school. Spending that time reading books, watching and acting out scenes from videos, practicing fine motor and language skills by drawing and building and describing action, playing, and using language to negotiate activity choices and peer interactions is more valuable than doing more worksheets. These hours are the child's prime time to have a richer experience than school alone provides.

Of course, if you work full-time, you'll respond to this sort of mandate with an exhausted sigh. Fair enough. There is only so much one person can do. But there's nothing wrong with recruiting help. A relative, a friend you can share care with, or an after-school care provider can provide some of this meaningful engagement after school. The important thing to understand is that opportunities for your child to learn occur at all kinds of times and don't stop when the paid personnel go home.

If this sounds onerous, try to look at it this way: This is no different from what any parent does to provide an enriching environment for any child. You may already agree with the philosophy that when the nanny goes home for the day or you pick your kids up at an extended-day program at school, they shouldn't just sit in front of the TV through dinner and until bedtime. The difference with your child who has autism is that you will need to learn special skills to understand how to fill this time. In Chapter 10 I'll explain how to acquire these skills by learning to work as a partner with therapists, teachers, and care providers.

Doing the Best for Your Child without Giving Up Yourself

Getting the diagnosis and swinging into action is surely going to change how your child spends his time. But what will it mean for *you*? You just read about all the things that will need to be arranged in your child's day. In Chapters 7 and 8 you'll read about specific services you're likely to need and how you will need to learn about those as well as communicate with service providers.

Where is all this time supposed to come from? What's going to have to give? Clearly you're going to have to do some reprioritizing. Here are some issues to examine as you consider what might be the best path to take.

"Do I Need to Give Up My Job?"

Sometimes on the day of the diagnostic assessment I am asked, "Does this mean I need to give up my job?" Probably not. Does it mean it will be harder to work a fifty- to sixty-hour week? Yeah; I've met very few sets of parents who work crazy hours *and* manage things with their child with autism *and* remain sane. (You *might* be able to swing it if you have a live-in grandma who is a retired speech therapist.) So how do you strike a balance?

The Designated Hitter

In most families, there is a "designated hitter." This is the parent who goes to bat for each and every doctor's appointment, drives to the therapy appointments, observes at school, and (seemingly) tirelessly attends IEP meetings. Sometimes parents manage to split these tasks up, but more often than not one parent carries things. Not surprisingly, this is often the parent who earns less income. Sometimes it is the parent with the more flexible work schedule—like a writer, artist, part-time academic, or employee of a large enlightened corporation with a human resources department that understands the need for flex-time and part-time work in situations like these. In some families we see, only one parent speaks English, and it's usually the breadwinner. By default, this parent is the interface with the outside world. I'd like to think that at least one segment of the population that has experienced less work stress since the advent of e-mail is parents like these—who can at least be in contact about their child whenever they can make time. If you are the "designated hitter" in your family, you are the one particularly vulnerable to all sorts of stress responses and need to make sure you observe some limits.

Setting a Time Line

One thing that helps some families is making a time line. It usually takes three to six months from the time you really get in gear setting up diagnostic appointments and assessments to get the show fully on the road. If you can take family leave, this is the time to consider it. Maybe you can take half-time family leave and still work half of the time. Maybe you stay a little more sane that way. (Only some of your life has changed, not everything.) Many families we see in our clinic have one parent take a year off. For example, teachers can, with relative ease, take off a year.

"Am I Bargaining?"

If you are in the process of deciding on time off, do it with some sense of the tasks you will be undertaking. One parent, very successful in her career, told me she was never going to work another day until her son lost his diagnosis. Her heart is in the right place. In this case, her son is one of those little guys who *might* lose his diagnosis. But who is she bargaining with? She has two full-time nannies, a well-established home program, a good preschool, and a child who is already doing a rather decent job of learning new things on his own. I'm not sure her intent not to work is so much related to what she needs to do for her son, as it is a talisman for her.

You may find yourself asking "What about the life I was meaning to have?" Since children with autism come into parents' lives during their child-bearing years, children with autism are also coming into parents' lives just when many are hitting their stride in the workplace. Even a little time off may mean you will feel you can no longer be at the top of your game. If this is you, there is no pat answer. It may or may not be strictly true that you are now destined to fail in meeting some of the goals you have idealized for yourself; but it sure may feel that way. There may be ways of changing which goals you meet, how fast you get there, or when you take them up again in earnest that you will need to work through. You may very well need some strong mentoring or therapy to clearly see all the issues you face in balancing your work with your autistic child. I meet many parents, particularly mothers, who feel that anything they want that would be designed to meet their own needs has become an unaffordable luxury. I would argue otherwise.

Helping Yourself So You Can Help Your Child

I'm sure you've heard flight attendants say "Put on your own oxygen mask before attempting to help others." There's a good reason for this dictate. In a life-threatening situation on an airplane, panic will be good for no one. If you can't breathe, you will be of no use to anyone. If your child's diagnosis throws you into a crisis of faith in yourself, your marriage, or your life goals, you will need help. Loss of work can feel like a loss of self. Loss of intimacy in your marriage can leave you alienated and unable to see your positive importance in critical relationships in your life. In a minute, we'll talk about the effects of having a child with autism on a marriage and on family and other sources of social support, but first we have to focus on you alone.

I remember a mother who was on a lecture panel with me some years ago. She had an eight-year-old, pretty severely involved nonverbal boy with autism. This was in Los Angeles, and she had done the de rigueur (at the time) forty hours a week of ABA/DTT therapy, taking her son to UCLA to Dr. Lovaas's clinic. He had shown some improvements, but not a world of change. She was glad she had done it. However, she exhorted the audience of infant development professionals to whom we were speaking: "Tell your moms to get themselves a therapist." She reviewed all the reasons she knew that other mothers she had met had not done this. Then she talked about how she and every mother of an autistic child she had met had been depressed during those first two years.

She was right, of course. All the changes you face are overwhelming. Being overwhelmed makes for helplessness and feelings of depression. If you blame yourself for having a child with autism, depression might seem like a suitable self-inflicted punishment. The trouble is, you did not cause this! Everything we know about the origins of autism suggests that no one can arrange things so that a child will be born with autism.*

There are very few psychotherapists (though the number is increasing) who specialize in the issues faced by parents raising a child with a serious disability. In the case of the woman I just described, she was able to return to a therapist she had seen off and on over the years for various other issues and who knew her well. A doctor who specializes in assessment of children with autism probably has psychotherapist colleagues who have expressed interest in seeing parents of children with autism. In my clinic we have a few such specialized therapists to whom we make referrals, as well as child psychiatrists (who all have had to do adult psychiatry training first) who have spent time with families in the Autism Clinic as part of their training.

---

*There is more about our understanding of what *does* cause autism in my book *The World of the Autistic Child* (see Resources at the end of this book).

Psychotherapeutic Help

I've been told many times, "If I had another seventy-five dollars a week to spend (which is what my weekly psychotherapy co-payment would be), I'd spend it on more speech therapy for my son." I'm not sure that would be the best investment. As I said earlier in this chapter, most children with autism need practice on their goals—in whatever area of learning—not a new curriculum, new drills, or new materials added to their treatment two to four times per week. That means that if you know what's going on in speech therapy, the time you spend reinforcing and practicing your child's goals with her is at least as important as another therapy hour. So—go for it; help yourself.

The work to be done in psychotherapy around dealing with a child with autism can usually be divided into two categories. One is how to cope, and you have two possible ways to tackle it: First, these days an increasingly popular therapy approach is something called *cognitive-behavioral therapy*, or CBT. With CBT, you basically list all your stressors (or at least your top ten) and then enumerate things you could do to ameliorate each objectively defined source of stress. This means that "having a child with autism" is not something that belongs on your list; some "operationally definable" part of what you find hardest about having a child with autism does belong there.

A very hard thing for you may be that your autistic child screams whenever you nurse your infant for more than five minutes or that he is at his crankiest at the time of day you must make dinner. Let's take the dinner example. Maybe you can hire a teenage babysitter each evening from six to seven while you make dinner. Even a twelve-year-old neighbor would be fine. You just need your child to be safe and moderately distracted from making demands on you to hand-feed him a snack—or whatever it is that makes him so cranky. Maybe you can start off just doing this for yourself two days a week and see if you feel at all relieved. Maybe having two nights a week when you order home-delivered take-out food will work better for you than a sitter. Whatever works for you. With CBT, the goal is to think of small ways to change your behavior or circumstances so you can respond to events in a less stressed-out fashion.

The second route to stress relief is through psychoactive medication. We know that psychotherapy accompanied by medicine is usually more effective than either is alone. (This, by the way means that a one-stop visit to a psychiatrist who puts you on an antidepressant, while not ineffective, is not likely to be the best you can do. To the extent that you take a "meds only" approach to self-treatment, you'll probably find yourself on higher rather than lower doses of whatever it is you are prescribed.) Many psychoactive medications these days have pretty low side-effect profiles if monitored responsibly, and the tranquilizers, like Valium, of days of yore that left you sleepy, spacy, and unable to operate a motor vehicle safely are not what we are talking about. Antidepressant or antianxiety medications are not addictive and can work equally well if you're dealing with a situation-specific stressor—like finding out your child is autistic—as well as depression, which may be an existing proclivity and which is acutely triggered by getting your child's diagnosis or trying to deal with stressful aspects of caregiving.

Coping with Grief

The other juggernaut, besides coping, is working through the stages of grieving for the loss of the child and the life you imagined. The first stage is the outcry, a disbelief that this is really true, that this could happen to you, the mother who wanted a perfect baby so much that you started to take prenatal vitamins while trying to get pregnant. Facing the sense of unfairness and dwelling on possible risk factors and dealing with what this shock means to future family plans are all part of coming to understand your initial response. Fathers more than mothers at this stage often can feel assaulted. Some respond by wanting to sue a doctor or "Big Drugs" (that some fearmongering websites will insist cynically put something in your baby's vaccines). The truth is that you did not plan to have this happen—but here you are. You will need help if you are not to get stuck in this initial "Why me?" stage of the grief cycle, where anger can become poisonous to everyone around you—including yourself.

After an initial period of outcry, the early fires can be quelled with the rains of denial. Some laypeople think "denial" is all bad—like "Wow, is *he* in denial!"—meaning that the person should know better. Denial, though, is a psychic defense mechanism that can serve the very healthy function of titrating the amount of distress you take in. For example, it's normal to worry that your child might not be ready for a regular kindergarten when she is five. It is less healthy to find yourself obsessed with the thought that she may never get married. One step at a time is all our CPU can handle without a system crash. Many people benefit from support in thinking about and prioritizing these concerns so every possible worry doesn't impinge at once.

Dealing with Intrusive, Unwanted Thoughts

Another expected part of the grieving process that many people can have a hard time dealing with is the emergence of unbidden, unwanted thoughts about the distress experienced. This can range from guilty fantasies about abandoning your family and starting a new life somewhere else to wishing something would happen to your child—or the child or a family member who is developing well. It's not that there is an evil person lurking inside you who really, truly wants these things or could or would act on impulses like these. It's that you're undergoing a mental process that is a type of steam release valve. Thoughts do not necessarily influence action, but it can be helpful just to have someone with whom you can talk about these things out loud. Talking can make what is unreal seem more unreal and therefore less threatening. Sometimes that releases enough steam to let the unpleasant unbidden images dissipate.

Working Through

Over time, some greater degree of acceptance comes to most parents of children with autism. This is not necessarily going to happen in the first year or two after a diagnosis, however. In my experience, parents of eight- to ten-year-olds are just getting to this point. At some point you can feel good that you've done what can be done. You (meaning your child) have accomplished some of the goals set out at age three or four or five. Some may remain unaccomplished—but somehow it doesn't feel as devastating now as you thought it would feel five years ago. Again, this is another healthy waystation on the road to recovering from the psychological impact of having a child who presents you with an unplanned journey. More long-term adaptations in your expectations for yourself, your career, your relationships with other people all have room to creep back into the agenda now. Some parents are transformed by their experiences and become special education teachers instead of general education teachers. Some lawyers start to focus on disability law instead of mergers and acquisitions.

Importantly, some people need more help (such as therapy) or simply more time coming to understand this new reality, and if you feel you are one of them, seek out that help for yourself—or you risk burning yourself out.

Using the *A* Word

"Doctor, can we not use the *A* word in front of him?"

Sure, fine. But why do you feel the need to ask? If the *A* was for "arthritis," would you say the same thing? Really, saying the name of a disability does not make it so. The word *autism*, used with a child with autism or PDD, or with a sibling, starts out as a black box—an empty black box. For your child with autism (when he gets to the point where he can understand) and his siblings, autism is what you tell them it is. It is all the things your child simply can't do (yet). While the symptoms of autism can make a child hard to live with, the extra work in caring for your child with autism is not some sort of punishment or result of bad family karma, as mothers and fathers from some cultures are told by their elders. Yes, it can be painful to say the word. Over time, though, being able to talk openly about your child's autism should desensitize you to the pain initially associated with the diagnosis. If you can talk about it with each other, the probability that you'll be able to develop a more mutual agreed-upon understanding of it and how to cope with it increases.

Stasis and Chronic Sorrow

Autism as a life stressor is really never over, but eventually everyone reaches some sort of stasis or way of living with autism. Humor helps. Adjusted expectations help. Support from others helps. How you employ these strategies and how you negotiate the rough patches is another point at which psychotherapeutic support can be of help. Even parents of children who have lost their diagnoses experience tremors when seeing their teen fail to perceive some obvious social cue. For other parents, these moments may come when you feel everything is going well and then, out of the blue, an afternoon with a cousin the same age as your child casts the differences into strong relief. Sometimes a reawakening of old feelings of injury occurs when someone talks about your child in front of you, not realizing that you are the parent (or realizing you are the parent). There are some days when it may seem that it can never be as easy to live with a child with autism as with a typical child. But you might need someone to remind you that autism has advantages over having a child that you worry is taking drugs, driving drunk, out there getting AIDS, or deciding he hates you so much that he moves out of your life and disappears. Life is full of trade-offs, and all people, all parents, need help and support to deal with them. This is to say that you, as the parent of a child with autism, will have some special issues—but you will never be alone in having stress.

Coping with the Stress of Special Caregiving

What are the special sources of stress you deal with as the parent of a child with autism? The hardest thing for parents of the youngest children may be watching how frustrated the child can become trying to communicate her needs and get her needs met. Early on, if not later on as well, many children with autism either lack verbal communicative

---

Accepting the Love That Your Autistic Child Can Give

In coping with a diagnosis of autism, parents experience a particular burden that is unique to autism, which is that the child is selectively impaired in social reciprocity. Although autistic children love their parents in their own ways, it's a different expression of need and affection from the parents' relationship with their other children and keeps parents reaching across some chasm to try to bridge the gap.

From what I've seen, I believe some degree of acceptance that the loving qualities of the relationship with the child with autism will always be different in some ways reduces stress and allows parents to increase the pleasure they take from their lives with their child with autism. Every moment that you expect something that isn't there, you may feel discouraged. But if you learn to appreciate the joys of your child's every accomplishment, and feel proud of where she's gotten to now—not just hopeful for where she may be in the future—you will likely feel less distressed and able to cope better. Essentially, parents who can see the child's differences as her "normal" seem to adjust best. Another approach that helps some families is seeing their children as "spies from God"—as I heard one sibling of a developmentally disabled adult say recently. For some families, caring for a child with autism well is an opportunity to rise to an important occasion.

---

means or don't use the language they do have to make a social connection. Through things like hand leading, language limited to the meeting of needs, and simply waiting to have needs anticipated, most children with autism and their parents eventually do arrive at some solution that allows a decrease in unhappiness and frustration. However, this communication can lack a sense of the loving dependence that allows parents to feel they are the mainstay of their child's emotional existence. Instead, children with autism tend to be more instrumental, relying on parents insofar as they are the ones who are seen as most efficiently meeting their needs.

A corollary of this is that the give-and-take of physical affection with a child with autism is much more often regulated by the child than the parent. If the child wants contact, parents give it; but, most often, when the child has had enough, she moves off, and the parent needs to learn to feel satisfied with that. One couple I know were initially distressed to realize that their toddler son did not seem to get excited (or even much notice) when Daddy came home from work in the way friends' children did. Rather than just moping and feeling bad about it, these parents devised a plan where the dad would call the mom on his cell phone when he was a couple blocks from home. The boy's mother would then begin to chat up his dad's arrival, practice hugging, and sound increasingly excited. Slowly, the little guy learned to recognize the sound of the garage door opening and to run up to his dad on his own.

Another special caregiving stress is seeing your child with agemates that you have known all their lives. I talk to many mothers who have had a sister or cousin who was pregnant at the same time. They start off with babies of the same age, and conversations are often about comparing the new things each has seen her baby do. The same thing happens with mothers who start off in the same prenatal exercise group, which progresses to a weekly Mommy and Me group: As your baby with autism starts to stick out—not watching the others, not joining in to watch a toy work or hear a story read, even avoiding the others—you, as the mommy this is happening to, will feel understandably distraught. (I hear the other side too—friends and sisters who want to help but are afraid that anything they say will be hurtful.)

Reaching out for support from your existing network is really important. Research shows that maintaining the fabric of the life you had before the diagnosis is more important to your longer-term well-being than forsaking it in favor of life as an autism-only mom or dad. You may have to make some leaps of faith to rely on the altruism and good will of others who don't experience what you are experiencing every day. Let these friends and family help you stay grounded. There is definitely an important place for what you can learn from autism support groups. But there's a downside too. Parents get competitive in subtle and not so subtle ways about who has the "best" therapist, the "most" hours, or the highest-functioning child. Every child with an autism spectrum disorder is different, and any such comparisons are likely to leave you finding something to feel worse about. If you find this happening to you, just stay away. In the next chapter, we will talk more about this in the context of things you'll encounter on the Internet—and how you navigate from the shoals of false hope.

Interdependence and Cooperation: No Man Is an Island

One of the serious pitfalls for parents of a child with autism is to feel that "no one but me" can be around the child. This can result in your turning a blind eye to the help that others proffer. Just because someone handles a situation differently from how you might does not mean your child is being irreparably damaged. All kids, including autistic kids, can be amazingly robust.

One of the difficult aspects of letting new treatment providers and caregivers into your child's life is managing your own anxiety that grows from a need to protect the child. The best example I can give of this is when a parent sees a new therapist work with her child the first time and doesn't like what she sees. Maybe the therapist *doesn't* have the right skill set. But maybe she is having a bad day. Maybe your child is having a bad day. Maybe the therapist is nervous about being scrutinized. Certainly it takes time for a relationship between child and therapist to develop. Don't cut out new people too quickly. Wherever you live, no matter how many resources you have at your disposal, you want to see if you "have a fish on the line" *before* you "cut bait" and prepare to cast your line again. The reason I am saying this now is that the more potential resources you turn away, the more boxed in you may find yourself. The more you have a network of others you can rely on, the less stressed you are likely to be.

The more people you have on your side, the better. Believe in the altruism of the human spirit. People want to help! If you now feel depressed and helpless about your child's situation, as most parents do for some or all or those first years, you may be looking at the world through dark lenses. Look for *where* you can get help and *who* is willing to help.

What about Your Marriage?

I know that having a child diagnosed with autism really strains a marriage. What may help is knowing that this stress is pretty universal. Even the best relationships are strained when hit with such a major life stressor. Sometimes it may feel like you can't love your child and your spouse at the same time. Wow! That would be really hard if it were true. How can you work things out so you don't emotionally (or actually) lose the other person closest to your child?

Special Risks: Blame, Polarization, Alienation

Each parent will have a different answer to the question of why you had a child with autism. Each parent is likely to express a different level of inherent optimism (or pessimism). The truth is neither you nor I nor anyone else knows all the factors that might have led to your child's difficulties. The truth is neither you nor I nor anyone else has a crystal-clear crystal ball and knows how things may turn out for your child. So, treating each other as if it's someone's fault is speculation. Acting like things will surely be worse if one of you doesn't believe good things might happen is also speculation. Nobody loves uncertainty. You both will need to live with significant uncertainty for an uncertain period of time. If you can face the reality that has become your parenting together, you'll probably feel stronger. Not that it's easy.

On top of its not being easy, parents are usually in separate places with respect to the grieving that follows the diagnosis. It can be hard to fully respect someone who seems to move through the coping more slowly than you have. The coping response you may feel critical of may not be new. If you've felt that your spouse was a "denier" when under stress in the past, it may seem that way now too. If you felt your spouse got stuck in anger in response to earlier stressors, that might be what's happening now. Thinking about things this way may help you see and feel what is going on with your partner. It may also reawaken past feelings about past traumatic events the two of you shared, reinflicting some of *that* psychic pain all over again. For goodness sake, see a counselor or a member of the clergy, or talk to a family member or friend you can trust to be neutral—and help you sort out your feelings.

Building In Protections:
Respite, Time Together, Preserving Intimacy

Research generally suggests that having a child with autism does nothing great for a marriage. I would say that half of the divorcing parents of autistic children I know admit there were problems before the child's diagnosis and that dealing with the child's special issues made things worse. The other half feel the diagnosis was more than what one or both could handle. I can think of very few couples over the years who have categorically stated that their child's condition had nothing whatsoever to do with the divorce. I know many unhappy couples who remain together in marriages now devoid of intimacy, too morally committed to the care of their child to leave the marriage. Studies show that loss of intimacy through spending one-to-one time mainly talking about the child is among the most problematic developments following a diagnosis.

What are the remedies? How about time away together? Preserve a "date" night. Have one family member, respite worker, or paid tutor that you can feel safe leaving your child with for a night a week or at least a night a month. I'm no fan of endless videos, but they have their place, and this is one of them. Talk about something else when you are away together. If you must talk about something to do with your child, make a rule that you'll start to talk about it only when you order dessert or when you are walking *out* of the movie.

If there are two people you can trust to leave your child with, go away overnight. It may be years before things feel as "in control" as they did before you started to focus on your child's special needs. Don't try to hold your breath until that day. Yes, routines for your child are important. Yes, consistency is important. Yes, dedicating financial resources to the best treatment you can devise is laudable. But one day or two days will not alter the course of your child's development. Maybe your home program on Monday will look lousy after Grandma was staying over Friday and Saturday night. Your child will rebound. You need a recharge too. Without recharging, you can't do your best by your child.

Preserving the Family: A Valuable Resource

Families can lose themselves in autism. Families who can't go to the mall on Saturday afternoons might feel like they can never go. They may never try going at 6:30 on a Wednesday, when it's pretty empty.

Families do better if they can come up with ideas to do things where the family feels whole and not atypical. The father of one family we worked with intensively in Hawaii wanted us to see his son at the beach. At the beach (where he was pretty water safe, like most Hawaiian three-year-olds), the fact that he didn't talk, understand language, or follow directions didn't look as remarkable bad as it did in his living room, when he was surrounded by five kinds of therapists. I really appreciated where this little guy's dad was coming from.

Sit down and make a list of things that each member of your family enjoys doing as a family. Which ones are hard to do with your child with autism along? Can you do them at a different time? Can you do them in a different place? Can you do them for not so long? Can you take someone along to help? If the answer to all these questions is no, maybe the answer is to do them without your child with autism. In the next section, we'll talk about why this is so important for siblings. It is also important for you, as parents raising this family together, to be like other families. To the extent that everything is taken over by autism, you are losing the battle for "normal"—which is where you hope all the work with your child will take you. Try to have some "normal" now.

Humor

Some families normalize their atypical experiences with their autistic children through humor. Dr. Stu Silverstein, with whom I wrote a book on the experience of siblings of developmentally disabled children, was the brother of a lower-functioning autistic boy a year and a half younger than him. He tells a story of growing up on the playgrounds of his housing project in New York, threatening to beat up other kids who called his brother a "retard." (Fortunately, Dr. Silverstein is a big strong fellow.) However, when he got to be a teenager, he began to tell other kids, "My brother's not a retard, he's a Republican!" It worked for him. Another family I know talks about how their son Arthur is their human GPS when they go on car trips. The line between making fun of someone and having fun with someone can be subtle, but achieving that balance can help.

What about the Other Kids?

For years I've had a real soft spot in my heart for siblings of children with autism. If you think *you* didn't ask to be the parent of a child with autism, remember that they certainly didn't ask to be the sibling of one. Sibling rivalry is bad enough. Battling a sibling on a playing field that is not level is even worse. What can compete with autism for parents' time, emotional, and financial resources? Let's think about protections that don't leave your nonautistic children thinking they are unworthy of having your love too.

The really good news is that siblings are incredibly empathic and altruistic. I have seen siblings as young as eighteen months old "help" an older autistic brother—get his bottle or his pacifier or give him a hug when he was crying. How do you capitalize on and nurture the altruism without quashing the individual identity of the typically developing sibling?

What Affects How a Child Experiences the Sibling with Autism?

The diagnosis of autism means different things for siblings of different ages and stages. It is different for brothers and sisters. Birth order matters too. There are no absolutes; but the research repeatedly demonstrates some general principles. Girls are more often involved in caregiving tasks alongside parents than brothers are. Older siblings are more often involved in caregiving tasks alongside parents than younger siblings are. Older sisters, as you might then expect, are those most expected to help. Older siblings take on teacher and co-parenting roles. Younger siblings do well when they are endlessly demanding of attention from their autistic sib—and can't accept "leave me alone" as an answer. For the child with autism, there are (different) benefits of having younger and older sibs. Many middle children I see do particularly well socially, other things being equal. In recent years, my clinic has seen a passel of nonidentical twins where only one has autism, and there seems to be a real value in having a constant companion to whom you (as the autistic child) are completely accustomed. I have also wondered whether these twin families with one typical and one special twin don't have something to teach us all about keeping any family normalized.

Teaching Siblings about Autism

What do you say—and what do you *not* say? Think of that black box I mentioned earlier. Make one for each brother and sister. If your autistic child does or doesn't do something because of his autism, tell his brother or sister that "autism" is the reason—"he didn't understand what I said," "he didn't answer," "he didn't look at me." Those observations go in the autism "box." Quite quickly, the sibling will get an idea of what is autism and what is not.

This means, of course, that not everything goes in the "autism" box. There are plenty of things any child should be expected to do. If your two-and-a-half-year-old can eat only in his booster seat at the table, then the same rule should be true for his five-year-old autistic brother who is developmentally more like two and a half. The two-and-a-half-year-old should hear the rule and see it being enforced—for him and for his brother. Autism is not an excuse not to do things you are old enough and smart enough to understand you need to do. As long as siblings see that rule in place, resentment is minimized to usual sibling rivalry levels.

Children with autism can be bad. If they are bad, they deserve the same consequences as a sibling at the same developmental level for a similar infraction. For a typically developing three-year-old who hits, a time-out in his room may be a good punishment that upsets him by isolating him and gives him an opportunity to internalize the mandate not to repeat the behavior that landed him there. You can't always use the same punishment with the child with autism, of course. Perhaps he *likes* being left alone in his room; then it is not a deterrent and in fact may be a reinforcer. His punishment may have to be an accompanied

---

Expectations

In Chapter 2 we discussed the pros and cons of "labeling" your child with people who can help her. In public, the diagnostic label can be used to manage expectations. At home, it can be used to manage expectations too. This means not substituting the word *infant* for *autism* or the word *incapable* for *autism*. A child with autism should be neither babied nor subjected to twenty-four-hour-a-day rules and restrictions. Each child needs to be treated with expectations appropriate for her developmental age—which will change with chronological age and with treatment. If you unconsciously stigmatize your child for her disability, and see her as incompetent, you will probably get what you wish for. Children, including autistic children, can rise to the occasion—*if it is expected of them.* If it is expected of them, your family will function better too.

time-out in plain view. The important thing is that siblings understand that everyone gets consequences for unacceptable actions.

Types of Sibling Coping

In *What about Me?: Siblings of Developmentally Disabled Children*, my colleague Stu Silverstein and I identified four subtypes of siblings based on our personal and clinical experiences. (Other people have since gone on to empirically characterize these types, too.) While no one child is going to fit perfectly into just one of these types, my guess is you will be able to identify the predominant type for each nonautistic sibling who is at least four or five years old. Understanding how your other kids might be responding to having an autistic sibling may help you prevent them from becoming overwhelmed and prevent the whole family from being thrown off course.

The Parentified Sibling

Older siblings, and especially sisters, can fall into acting like parents with respect to their sibling with autism. This happens quite naturally to older siblings in a single-parent family and in blended families where the child with autism comes along years later in a second marriage. Parentified six-year-olds hold their brother's hand as they walk down a hallway—without being asked. They carry the diaper bag. During diagnostic interviews they clarify exactly where certain of their sib's echolalic TV talk comes from—as they spend just as much time watching the same videos.

The good news is that parentified children often grow up to be "helpers" in disproportionate numbers: pediatricians, teachers, speech therapists, and so on. The bad news is that they may feel as if their sensitivity, empathy, and helpfulness are the main reasons they are loved and that their own accomplishments (like really good grades) aren't as richly rewarded as they might be if their parents weren't so occupied with their sibling's issues.

The Superachiever

The focus of superachievers is to gain parental kudos not through success with their autistic sib but rather through their own successes. One such young woman recently received a young filmmakers award for a short film about growing up with a brother with autism. The superachieving sibling is not only excellent in his own right but also makes up the GPA for the sibship as a whole. This is the child who feels that he or she can't be noticed too much. Two sisters, six and two years old, on their way to superachieverhood, changed outfits hourly (including fairies, ballerinas, Disney princesses Belle or Jasmine) to distract in-home therapists from their three-year-old autistic brother, who anyone could see was not nearly as well dressed as they.

Having a superachieving child can be a tremendous relief. While you know you did not cause your child's autism, having a child who is better than average restores confidence in parents that they *can* make good babies. Being motivated by a drive for parental love and attention is not a bad thing either, but if it's not as gratifying as you wish, or you seek to be a superachiever and, in your own mind, fail, you set yourself up for going through life with an unrealistic, perhaps obsessive drive for perfectionism.

The Withdrawn Sibling

Life with an autistic sibling is more than some kids can handle, especially those born after the autistic sibling and maybe even more so for those born so soon after that it was not yet known that their older brother or sister had a difficulty. This child may never have had her moment in the sun, when she was the center of the parental universe. I worry about a six-week-old in a baby carrier, trudged along to the diagnostic assessment of a two-and-a-half-year-old brother. I really worry about the baby of the mother who came to my clinic having put off her planned C-section for two days to have the diagnostic assessment for that baby's older brother. The withdrawn sibling comes to my clinic and busies herself in the corner of the play room, so isolated and self-isolating that I begin to wonder if she might be "on the spectrum" too. Then when I talk to this sort of child and draw her out, I discover a delightful child with a great imagination and wonderful words to describe her inner life. (I carry on the bottom of my IBM ThinkPad a "My Little Pony" sticker presented to me by such a little girl. It is my good-luck talisman that assures my ThinkPad will not be confused with someone else's as it goes through airport security.)

The Acting-Out Sibling

Some siblings can't handle the stress added to their family life by their autistic brother or sister. They can't figure out how to compete successfully for their share of the parental pie the way the parentified or superachieving child can. They can't create a safe place to live more or less alone as the withdrawn child may. Most often this type of sib is a boy. Sometimes this sib has his own mild neurodevelopmental issues like a learning disability, an attention deficit disorder, an anxiety disorder, or a tendency toward oppositional defiant behavior. When young, this child may see his autistic sib as an easy victim. If the only parental attention he can get is negative, he may go for that if he feels neglected. You, of course, are the overwhelmed parent and not neglecting him on purpose, so his behavior can feel like salt rubbed in a wound. This child needs more time alone with you. As we'll discuss in the next section, there's a variety of strategies you can consider to make your family dynamic work more smoothly.

Striking a Balance between Autism and Everything Else

Loving each child is something parents do naturally. But kids need different kinds of love. In the early years after diagnosis, much of your love for your child with autism is expressed in what you do *for* her. For your other children, it may be best expressed by what you do *with* them.

Find a way to make each child king or queen for the day. Certainly this should include birthdays. If your daughter is nine, nine-year-old girls typically want only other girls at their party. They might want to string beads or paint toenails. Your daughter should be able to do this free of concern that her autistic brother is a bead eater or that the carpet might be ruined if a certain someone started spilling nail polish everywhere. If your son of the same age wants to go with buddies to Disneyland on his birthday, he should be untroubled by the fact that his autistic brother wants to do only the spinning teacups or is toasted for the day after more than a fifteen-minute wait in any line.

Even better are regular opportunities where your typically developing child can count on your being there to cheer her to develop onward and upward: A Mommy and Me class, soccer games, or a class play or recital come to mind. If needed, leave the child with autism home if there is risk he'll rain on his sib's parade by taking you away from the scene when his sibling scores a goal, says her lines, or gets his turn to play. Usually, there is no way for the autistic sib to know what he's missing. There may be your guilt that, of course, you'd be taking him along if he wasn't autistic—but he is. It's a trade-off. Is having him come along and moan miserably in the parking lot worth your daughter being onstage looking for you and not seeing you as she says her lines? If you can do both, that will of course be the best. Many families can't always do that, so be prepared to make some trades where your child with autism might have to yield the right of way to siblings.

Moving from Getting Your House in Order to Dealing with the Outside World

Autism requires you to reshape your sense of self, your marriage, and your family life. Yes, there's a lot to work through. Strive to keep it normal. You will not be able to do that every day and in every way, but if you can set your sights on living like everyone without a child with autism does, you will be better equipped to do your best for the child with autism. In the next chapter, we will start to talk about how you figure out exactly what to do for your child and where, exactly, to look for the best possible providers and services.

FIVE

Becoming an Informed Consumer

GETTING YOUR "PERSONAL BEST"
IN SERVICES AND PROVIDERS

In the world of sports, when athletes achieve a "personal best," it means they are improving on their own best performance. In getting help for your child, you'll be reaching for a "personal best" of sorts: An understanding of what your child specifically needs will assure you are an informed consumer. Part III will help you build on what you learned from your child's assessments so you can prioritize his treatment needs. There are more really high-quality services to choose among for a child with autism than ever before and more providers with an appreciation of how important individualizing a treatment plan is. There are also more people out there hawking their autism "wares." Some know less than they think they do and earnestly offer a guaranteed fix based more on conviction than, say, science, solid theory, or common sense. Other "hawkers" are downright, cynically, okay with making a quick buck off anyone who chooses of his own free will to buy what they are selling. This chapter will help you become a discriminating consumer. I'll show you how to tell which treatment approaches are backed up by the "hardest" science—both established treatments and new developments—and which are essentially snake oil. Add to that some guidelines for choosing the best providers, and you have a clear map for implementing a treatment plan custom designed to benefit your child.

The Web: A Travel Guide to Autism's Superhighway

On the day I sat down to start this chapter, I began by going to Google and typing in "autism." There were 5,920,000 hits. The first two were sponsored links—folks who'd like you to give them money so they can investigate the aspects of autism most important to them. Listed fourth was the Autism Society of America, the oldest and largest parent support network and clearinghouse for information on autism in the United States and probably the world. It wasn't until I got to the seventh link that I found the website for the National Institutes of Health—the single best source of information on the "real" science of autism in the world. I had to scroll down once to get to that NIH link. Then, on the second page, under the sixth listing, cryptically entitled "Autism Information Center—NCBDDD, DCD," I found the portal to all that the CDC (Centers for Disease Control and Prevention) has to say to parents about autism; and they think they are doing a good job of getting their information "out there." In the several months between the time I started this chapter and finished this book, the information on autism on the Web has mushroomed to 21,600,000 hits. I can guarantee you we have not learned four times more about autism than we knew several months ago, but a quick trip to the Web might lead you to that conclusion. Caveat emptor: Buyer beware.

What if you, as a parent, had gotten bogged down going through the sites one by one as listed? You might well never have made it to the sources most researchers, doctors, and parents who've been around the block with this stuff a couple of times depend on. Gold mining is a good analogy for what it's like to find valuable information on autism from the Web. It's a tiny fraction of what's there, and you've got to sift through a lot of dirt to get to it. If you learn anything from this chapter, it will be how to recognize the real thing when you find it. All that glitters is not gold.

Being Web-Wise

What criteria should be applied to your sifting and sorting? There are no keywords I can think of that help me skirt the sites that send worried parents of a maybe-autistic child or parents of a newly diagnosed child in a less than useful direction. I want to help you avoid the crying-over-spilt-milk websites and focus on the let's-get-to-work websites. Later in this chapter we'll deal with "Steering Clear of the Shoals of False Hope." For now, suffice it to say that a large amount of what you can read about on the Web focuses on raising your level of paranoia about everything your child ever ingested, everything you ever ingested, the air we breathe, which Big Brother conspired to make these things a problem, and which other Big Brother is now protecting him. This is not to say that autism doesn't come from somewhere (we'll also go at sorting these facts from fiction in the next chapter), but that once autism is a reality in your life, much of what you can do to help comes from developmental, educational, and behaviorally based interventions.

As you travel the Web in search of hope, keep the purchase of used cars in mind: Would you approach sponsored links with skepticism? I hope so. Would you use common sense? (For instance, do you think a ten-year-old Mercedes is likely to be in better shape than a ten-year-old Fiat?) I hope so. Are you responding to marketing? (For instance, do you prefer the websites with the "preowned, certified" Mercedes to the ones with the "used" Mercedes?) Who wouldn't prefer a "preowned, certified" car to a "used" one? But, are you paying for spit and polish or a better car if you buy a "preowned" one?

The easiest criterion to apply to judging the veracity of autism treatment websites is that if something seems too good to be true, it probably is. If you can't see why something should work, maybe it doesn't. If the reason something is supposed to be better is that it costs three times as much as something else that does the same thing, maybe the main difference between the two things is that one is more expensive. If you can't see a difference other than cost, maybe that's the only difference. We're not buying Prada here.

Where's the Good Stuff?

Ideally, what you are looking for is information on the Web that is peer reviewed. This means a group of people who have well-regarded expert credentials in understanding autism have put their heads together and reached a consensus on the state of the art about their topic of focus. These are professionals who publish in scientific journals reviewed by others in their field, professors at major universities, accepted as experts in court hearings—people who are not going to make a dime based on whether you believe them or not. They are not autism's Johnny-come-lately types, who have suddenly and serendipitously cured autism by accident while treating some heretofore unrelated problem.

In addition to snake-oil salesmen, there are well-meaning parents who just don't get it but think they do, think what worked for them will work for everybody, and want to tell you what to do with *your* child: Recently, a journalist from a respected, peer-reviewed journal sent me a YouTube link and asked what I thought of the parent demonstrating a "treatment" he'd come up with for his child. This link had had hundreds of hits and boasted four stars, a psychobabble voice-over, and one unhappy-looking little autistic seven-year-old being trained to follow a bouncing ball.

With those caveats in mind, know that the Web can be a valuable resource for both global and local sources of expert help. For good, up-to-date, evidence-based information on autism and autism treatment, look for sites supported by the:

- National Institutes of Health (NIH)
- National Institute of Mental Health (NIMH)
- National Institute of Child Health and Human Development (NICHD)
- Centers for Disease Control and Prevention (CDC)
- World Health Organization (WHO)
- American Academy of Child and Adolescent Psychiatry (AACAP)
- American Academy of Pediatrics (AAP)

You can reach these websites by searching under "autism" paired with the name of the organization. These websites contain peer-reviewed content that may be a bit dry, a bit reductionistic for the more sophisticated reader. But—they don't lie. So they are a good place to start. Get the lay of the land. If you're looking for information on a particular autism treatment—say craniosacral therapy—and you find that none of these "science-based" sites endorse it, you know to be skeptical of sites that tout that it is the latest, greatest treatment for all sorts of autism problems from poor eye contact to lack of language—to a bad back. These sites I've just listed are kept pretty up to date, and most note when they were posted or last revised. Anything that's too new (untested) for one of these sites may well lack any science (or scientific reasoning).

What's Science?

Does that sound like a trick question? All the term *science* refers to is that which derives from logic rather than faith and hope. But that's not enough to tell you what constitutes a valid treatment for autism. How will you know one when you see it?

First, you're likely to see the words *evidence-based* tacked in front of certain treatments, so it's worthwhile to understand how things get to be referred to that way. In fact, if you're to understand how to interpret the "research" claims you'll encounter everywhere, you'll need to "unpack" the concept of evidence-based treatment.

Unfortunately, there is not enough of the ideal kind of data out there for us to know what exactly is best to do for a particular child with autism. (If cancer research was in this kind of shape—well, there would be a lot fewer cancer survivors.) Instead, in the field of autism treatment, we have to rely on different tiers of evidence: Basically, there are five types of evidence we tend to rely on. As we go down the successive tiers, the evidence can get shakier, so that's when it will be really important for you, as buyer, to beware. Let's start with the best.

Empirical Evidence

The best evidence is *empirical* evidence—you compare two treatments in a fair way, and in the future you rely on the treatment that came out on top in the comparison. (For example, is an aspirin or a sugar tablet better for a headache? The answer: an aspirin. Therefore, we can say that based on empirical evidence, most people would be better off taking an aspirin than a sugar tablet when they have a headache.) This sounds straightforward enough until you begin to think critically about what needs to be taken into account when you make a fair comparison of two treatments. People like psychometricians, biostatisticians, and epidemiologists spend their lifetimes arguing about which "fair" is the fairest of them all. Here are some key guidelines you might think about when you read about empirical research that reached one conclusion or another about an autism treatment.

- Were equivalent groups of individuals with autism compared?
- Did the groups studied represent all kinds of individuals with autism (or at least the one for whom you are interested in finding effective treatment)?
- Does it seem like there were enough individuals studied to justify each conclusion?
- Could something else that wasn't studied just as easily (or more easily) explain the treatment's outcome?
- Were the individuals tested both before and after treatment on the thing it was hoped the treatment would change in the first place? (For example, a diet change that clears up diarrhea is welcome to any parent of an excessively poopy child, but what about when one mother claimed that a treatment for diarrhea turned out to help her son's language development? If you can't figure why these two things would be linked—then maybe they really aren't.)
- Are there longer-term studies to show that any treatment benefits endured after the treatment was stopped?
- Are there any indications of who did best and who changed the least from this treatment?

Empirically Based Comparative Theory

The next best evidence comes from findings that are consistent with existing empirical evidence—even though the specific topic at hand may not itself have been subjected to empirical comparison. (For example, is an aspirin and a cup of hot tea better for a headache accompanied by congestion than an aspirin alone? Since hot liquids tend to loosen congestion, we might reasonably assume that the former treatment is better, even though no medical journal has likely ever published a paper on the effectiveness of aspirin plus tea versus aspirin alone for treating a head cold.)

Broader Theory-Based Evidence

A third tier of evidence we often must rely on is whether an empirically untested treatment is consistent with widely accepted theory. In devising autism treatments, we have had to draw on lots of different kinds of theory. We'll talk about three kinds of theory: behavioral theory, child development theory, and social policy theory.

Only one method of *behavioral theory* has been applied and tested in comparative groups of children with autism and rises to the level of evidence being described as empirical. This is discrete trial training (DTT). Much of the rest of what is done in the name of behavioral theory with autistic children is just that—theory. Behaviorists often go about gathering evidence differently from other types of investigators: Behaviorists often study cases involving a single child at a time and replicate a predicted finding *within* a case rather than *between* cases the way folks that compare groups are essentially doing. These single-case-at-a-time approaches are informative, but many consider them better for theory *testing* than for theory *confirming* because one child with autism can be so different from another.

Theory from the field of child development is often applied to designing autism treatments whether we realize it or not: Studying typically developing children has told us a lot about the order in which abilities emerge. Much of what educators do in treating autism is to follow the order described in the developmental literature but use special methods of helping those abilities develop. In fact, educators mainly rely on behavioral theory for their methods, though not necessarily just DTT, the most empirically based of the behavioral methods. (For example, when a teacher praises a child for a performance she hopes will be repeated, breaks a task down into components and teaches them one at a time, or calls on the child who is raising his hand quietly, she is, in turn, using positive reinforcement, task analysis, and differential reinforcement—though she may not call them that.) When theory-based practices are adopted, the theories being applied are not necessarily mutually exclusive.

Another way that theory informs treatment practice for children with autism is through *social policy*—which is essentially another kind of theory. Social policy can reflect all sorts of socialization practices aimed at inculcating values to make society better in agreed-on ways—like recycling, eating healthy food, or including special education pupils in general education classes. While there is some *empirical* evidence supporting inclusion as a treatment for autism, it actually has more support as a social policy. This is because it has mainly been studied empirically, in just certain kinds of children with autism (higher-functioning ones) and only in certain kinds of carefully supported educational settings (like lab schools), and even the people who do the research realize you can't include just anyone, anywhere. Mainly, the impetus to include is supported by the theory that we will be a better society for it—that, for example, nonautistic peers will learn to practice altruism and tolerance.

Clinical Acumen and Experience

Another way that we say we "know" how to treat autism is through clinical acumen and experience. In the field of medicine, this is often the fallback position when there are no specific studies to recommend one practice over the other. Basically, we depend on a doctor who has experience with lots of similar cases to use her cumulative memory as a database and more or less run the statistics mentally. How good is this? It can be very good, or it can be very problematic. An experienced clinician's best asset is (1) knowing the research and (2) knowing what has happened to her patients or pupils over time as a result of different treatments and maturation. There is almost no longitudinal (long-term) research on autism treatments right now. The best information we have about long-term effects of treatment for autism is all in the heads of a small number of clinicians who have followed the same autistic children for ten to twenty years. Unfortunately, there are not enough of us. Another problem is that many people who diagnose autism don't see the same children regularly over time. Treatment providers such as educators are more likely to fall into that category. The education literature, however, does not tell us where the various kinds of children with autism who attended a preschool class are when they are eighteen years old. Part of the reason we lack such data is that educators tend to specialize in preschoolers, school-age kids, high-schoolers, and so on. Most lose track of kids they worked with as they move on. This means that someone who treats only preschoolers may not personally be particularly well informed about what happens to children who receive their treatment as they have grown up—so take anything they say about long-term treatment outcomes with a grain of salt. It is only human nature to believe that the treatment you give is the most effective one available. However, it is a reasonable assumption that a treatment that is much more effective in the short term will be better in the longer term than treatments that have been less effective in the short term. Be mindful, however, of the fox-minding-the-henhouse effect: By this I mean that folks who say the treatment they are "selling" just happens to be better than anything else do have a bit of a vested interest in whether or not you go with their treatment.

Anecdotal/Case-Based Findings

The final type of evidence we will talk about is what I consider the softest. Any conclusion based on just one seemingly amazing case needs to be replicated carefully with other cases studied in a similar way. A good example would be the one I mentioned earlier—the assertion that clearing up an autistic child's diarrhea helps his language development too. When this assertion was tested in a controlled fashion, the findings disappeared.

This does not mean that all single-case findings are hooey. One important research tool is what behaviorists often do, which is something called *single-case designs*: Unlike theoryless but hopeful assertions that arise from thin air, behaviorists will start with a theory and a prediction of what they expect to find. This really allows the single-case-findings behaviorist's reach to ring true in a way that is logical and quite different from the cure-diarrhea-and-you'll-help-language-development assertion.

It's human nature to want to create a miracle for your child if he seems beyond your help. How can parents not want to rescue their own child when that child feels increasingly lost? Unfortunately, some parents who feel this way also have rather histrionic personalities and cope with their terrible feelings of loss and helplessness by laying claim to a miracle they have personally wrought.

There are many examples of this among the things you can read about autism on the Web. One that comes to mind is the example I have already talked a bit about—the diarrhea–autism link—which came out of one child's diagnostic testing to find a cause for his gastrointestinal difficulties: This is the secretin story, a great case example in understanding how the horse of hope led the cart of science.

As an autism scientist who has enough to do reading journals, writing books, and assessing children, I blissfully don't have much time for blarney. So, I first heard about secretin when it hit the left-hand column of the front page of the *Wall Street Journal* as the pot of gold at the end of one mother's brave journey—wherein she had serendipitously discovered that a compound used in medical testing for her child's chronic diarrhea was in fact a cure for autism. (The trading initials of this pot-of-gold manufacturer were, of course, also in this *Wall Street Journal* article.) Turns out, about five years and I don't know how many millions of dollars and dashed hopes later, this mom's kid had actually never had a comprehensive diagnostic assessment for autism and had started an ABA program at the same time he started secretin—but, she asserted, it was the secretin that was making all the difference. Following up on the publication of this column, secretin created quite a hullabaloo. Even the parents who had signed their children up for a rigorous double-blind study of secretin at a university medical center and who turned out to be in the placebo group thought secretin had helped. (This time the secretin findings were reported in the *New England Journal of Medicine*—which, to be fair, has editors who probably know as much about the stock market as *Wall Street Journal* editors know about medical research.) Hope springs eternal.

If, after the fact, someone claims to have significantly improved some aspect of a child's autism by, say, some dietary intervention I have never heard of before, I ask myself at least four sets of questions:

1. When they made this change in diet, what did they expect? This? Anything? Something completely different?
2. Was anything started around the same time that could account for changes and might be a more conventional explanation for any change?
3. Does the change, whatever it is, seem as notable to me as it does to the teller? Can I measure it on any test? Does the thing that changed still seem like a big problem?
4. Do I know of any existing empirical evidence or theory that could explain what is said to have changed?

This is how I start to feel out placebo effects.

Placebo Effects

How will you detect a placebo effect if you encounter one? It can be fairly hard for a parent. It's a bit easier for me—though not because I know everything there could be to know about all this. As a parent, one is in the netherworld of tea leaves and fortune cookies. (I live in San Francisco, so I know where to go to buy a fortune cookie that will say whatever I want.) As with fortune cookies, it's possible to see your kid in almost anything you read about autism. If there's a treatment that worked for that child you're reading about, why shouldn't it work for your child too? What could it hurt? How could you live with yourself if this proved to be the silver bullet and you passed it by? The pull of your emotional brain wanting to see the similarities is very likely going to be stronger than the pull of your rational brain saying, "Whoa, maybe not."

So why is it easier for me? Aside from the self-evident truth that the child is yours and not mine, I'm peering into the opposite end of the lens. An example: I sit in my clinic as one parent after another comes in and says, "We've gone ahead and started trying the gluten-free, casein-free (GFCF) diet. Read so much about it on the Internet. Ordered the rye bread from Canada and everything. We're all doing it." I say, "So how's it going? What got you to go for it? Seen any improvements?" Then I may hear one of the following: "Well, actually nothing behaviorally, but his cheeks aren't ruddy all the time, and the chronic diarrhea's cleared up." Another parent might say, "He started talking the week we got him off the gluten products!" Another: "Eye contact is *much* better." Other parents tell me that the GFCF diet has had a marked impact on their child's hyperactivity. I say to myself, "Wow! What drug do we have in the whole field of medicine that's good for loose stools, delayed language development, poor eye contact, and hyperactivity? Aspirin? No! . . . I know! A placebo!"

As a parent, of course, you have no way to get the view of this that I get. Thinking that a correlation means causation is quite understandable if you're working with only one data point (one child). Parents of children with autism also tend to be guilt magnets. There are many websites where you can read that if the GFCF diet isn't working, you just aren't getting it right yet. I've been asked how to get to McDonald's during the lunch break at my clinic—because only McDonald's has gluten-free French fries. Really? It's been pointed out to me that other restaurants might be using their deep fryers for breaded foods as well as fries and some breading might float off and stick to the fries, messing everything up.

Parents of the youngest children with autism are particularly vulnerable to placebo effects—first, because there's a lot of developmental improvement going on anyway, even if you fear there's not; and second, because parents of the youngest children have had less (or no) time yet to see response to proven interventions, so there is nothing against which to gauge the magnitude of any perceived changes.

Selecting Services

Okay, the late-night sessions of crawling all over the Web are over—for now. You get the idea. You need to get started getting things in place for your child. Your engine is revving, but in some ways you feel you're revving in neutral. If you put it in gear, you might go in the wrong direction. What if you choose the wrong school? The wrong class? The wrong teacher, therapist, or tutor? Will you make things worse? Will you lose precious time? How critical is each decision you need to make? How do you set priorities?

The first thing to remember is that we have no evidence that there is one best way to treat a child with autism. What you choose to do will depend on what your child's capacities are right now, what kinds of behavioral challenges may be blocking the road to learning, and how hard you can push. What this boils down to is that there is no one best way for any one child. There are always multiple routes you can take to get there—wherever "there" will be for your child. I believe it's the ambiguity of not knowing the "there" you're headed for that makes many parents seek certitude in the first treatments they go after. This means you may want the "best" speech therapist, more hours of ABA, and as much one-to-one everything as you can get. Okay, it's reasonable to feel that way. I understand where it's coming from. But the law is designed to ensure an equitable distribution of resources. This is why the law says your child is entitled to an "appropriate" program—not the most expensive program. (In America, we tend to equate expensive with better.) Right away, many parents get into a battle stance with the system, thinking that fighting for "more" or "more expensive" is better or more right for their child. Sometimes it is. Sometimes it is not necessarily so. Let's develop some criteria so that you can feel you know "enough" when you see it—and don't drive yourself crazy always thinking "more" would be better.

How Do You Know If a Provider Is *Right* for Your Child?

Not everyone can do everything for anyone. No one can do something for everyone. In the field of psychological research, we call investigation of these principles *the study of individual differences*. What you will learn is that your child will do best when there is a match between who she is and the people who are there to help her. This is not just a matter of good and bad or even good and better therapists. It's about how well your child clicks with a particular treatment provider.

Components of a Great Service Provider

A service provider is anyone who provides services to your child. Most often, service provision is tiered: You may deal with a special education director who is incredibly knowledgeable, has been to every major conference or gotten every type of training you've read about, and knows autism specialists you've read about on a first-name basis. It's a great start! But who works for her? Who will be hands on with your child?

You may select a nonpublic agency to provide an ABA/DTT program for your child. The director of the agency may have gotten his or her PhD in Ivar Lovaas's lab. Great! But who works for her? Who will be hands on with your child?

Typically, the head of a special education department or a nonpublic agency or school that provides services for children with autism has tiers of people beneath him or her. We would like to believe that the best of those at the top can and do choose people who can be just as good to join the ranks below them. This is usually, mostly true. But there are pressures to do otherwise. Public education is subject to hiring based on credentials, seniority, unions, nondiscrimination policies—all sorts of factors that can do relatively little to reassure parents that a service provider will be the right match for their child.

Nonpublic agencies for autism treatment, as we will discuss in the next section, are rather the opposite—the Wild West. Pretty much anyone can hang out a shingle. (I was an expert in a lawsuit recently where it turned out the principal of the agency had a bogus online bachelor's degree—but *was* trained as a massage therapist.)

No one provider will always be the best for anyone who comes her way—no matter how good she is with one particular child you may know or have heard about. And no parent, of course, has unlimited choices of providers—for all sorts of reasons. But don't talk yourself into thinking you have no choice at all or that a choice being presented to you is good just because it is available to you. You do have choices, and you can keep a general formula in mind that will help you organize your thoughts and observations when you meet someone who could end up working directly with your child; see the diagram on this page.

The Best Treatment Providers

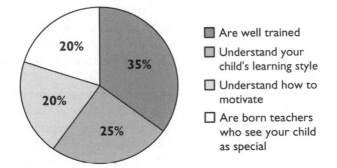

- Are well trained
- Understand your child's learning style
- Understand how to motivate
- Are born teachers who see your child as special

As you can see, my best guess of what makes a good service provider has to do with many things. No one component is everything. The key components are all critical. These are the key factors. When they are *not* there, they will likely result in an eventual change in providers—which, I think we can agree, everyone wants to avoid if possible.

Good Training

The most vital factor is good training. Good training has two key dimensions: First, the provider should have expertise with whatever technique he is using with your child—be it Floortime or math tutoring. If he is not an expert yet, he should have access to good supervision by someone who is significantly more expert. He should be on a learning curve that you can see the longer he works with your child. If a service provider is not an expert, you should have access to the supervisor yourself—for your training. (When it comes to working with their child, parents should not rely on supervision from twenty-year-old undergraduates or paraprofessional aides with an two-year degree and twelve units in education and child development.) Much of what needs to be done day to day, moment to moment with autistic children is to provide consistency, learning opportunities, and developmentally appropriate instruction. Then, it's practice, practice, practice.

At the most hands-on level, a classroom aide or a home tutor provides most of the one-to-one instruction a child with autism gets when he gets one-to-one. These providers are essentially technicians. I don't expect them to know much about autism—and neither should you. They will very likely not know what the suspected causes of autism are. They will very likely not be up on how double-blind medication trials work. They will very likely have no real way to know whether your child has Asperger syndrome and not autism. If they think they know, fine. You don't need to evaluate them on that basis anyway. What a service provider doing mainly one-to-one work should have is expertise in how to structure moment-to-moment activity. (To be fair, the geneticists, psychopharmacologists, and diagnosticians who *do* know about these things are unlikely to understand the nitty-gritty of treatment.)

How will you know if your nitty-gritty treatment provider is competent? For one thing, she should not seem like she is making it up as she goes. She should be able to articulate how her actions are intended to encourage some behaviors and decrease others. She should be able to see your child as having similar capacities to those that you, the expert on your particular child, know are there. Someone who feels your child is less able will expect too little. Someone who thinks that your child has capacities that have not yet reasonably had an opportunity to develop (as the people who used to do facilitated communication asserted) is not in tune with your child either.

The Ability to Apply General Knowledge to a Particular Child

Good training is just the first 35% of what you need to find in a really good service provider. The next 25% or so is that individual's ability to apply the knowledge to your child. There are two major dimensions to this too: Children with autism are all different because the specific symptoms of autism that handicap each the most differ, as well as because of differences in developmental level. Someone who has worked well with verbal autistic children may not excel in the same way with nonverbal children. Someone who is great at doing discrete trials may not have the skill set to teach reading just as well. The second dimension is the ability to respond to an individual child's autistic learning style (which we will discuss more in Chapter 6). This means a provider needs to have a sense of how visual versus auditory the presentation of teaching materials should be. The provider should have a sense of what kinds of inputs might overwhelm the child and interfere with an ability to learn. (For example, for some children this could be background noise, the nearness of others, physical contact, the size of the space used for teaching, and so on.) The provider should have a sense of what she can rely on for recall—such as visual images, music, rote auditory memory, or following physical routines. Many treatment programs build in methods and content that are synergistic with autistic learning styles, which is great. However, a really good provider, no matter the method being used, should have a sense of how to detect these strengths in your child and use them to help him shine—and feel successful in his learning.

The Ability to Motivate and Engage the Child

The third major factor that comprises the profile of a really good direct service provider is the ability to teach in a way that motivates and engages the child. I'll give that about a 20%. There are many tangible as well as less tangible factors here. Are the curriculum materials fun? Does the provider make them as fun as possible? Think about the Dr. Seuss story where Sam-I-Am finally gets the protagonist to eat green eggs and ham. He liked them! That required an ability to turn something initially judged to be completely yucky into something acceptable. A lesson for us all! A tutor or aide more concerned with protecting her dignity may not be the right fit for some children. I'm not saying you should look for clownlike service providers—rather ones that motivate your child. For many children with autism, it's knowing what's happening next that's motivating. For others it's about being able to exercise control in the teacher–pupil relationship—like finding a way for the child to ask for breaks, choices, or a specific reinforcer. A service provider who is well trained and is providing well-tailored intervention but just can't be interesting will have a hard time teaching your child as much as one who understands the motivation piece. (When I encounter this problem with a provider, I always think of my statistics professor in graduate school, who was supercompetent— he'd invented some of the statistics he taught, and he knew what we needed to learn next—but had a hell of a time making it interesting enough to keep anyone awake except through fear.)

If you've been keeping track, you noticed that we've accounted for only 80% of what makes a good service provider so far. At least 20% is a bunch of little things, such as a tutor who really loves your child and goes beyond the call of duty, knitting him something for his birthday, or offering to babysit while you and your spouse go away for your anniversary. Part of it is that the service provider is just a born teacher. This might be a tutor who, although young and relatively inexperienced, can be a great "energy match" for your child: Some children who are low energy do better with someone who can be calm too. Sometimes it's vice versa. Again, you, the expert on your particular child, can best imagine what will work out for your child. There are other factors too that we might just call "chemistry"—maybe your child responds inexplicably well to large guys, women who wear perfume on their necks, or people who have fluffy hair. These intangibles are great to have—though not to be confused with the key factors that contribute to what makes a teacher, therapist, tutor, or aide a great match for your child.

Finding the Best Providers: Is It a Buyer's or a Seller's Market?

Okay. I won't keep you in suspense. It's a seller's market.

There are many more people seeking good-quality appropriate services for children with autism than there are services to go around. This is true of the public education programs. It is true of the best nonpublic agencies and schools. It's true of the best therapists. Either they don't have openings, don't take your insurance, don't take kids the age your kid is going to be next month, or have a six-month waiting list.

How do you get noticed? How do you get your choice of the good service providers you now know how to identify? There are two answers. First, you know what you need for your child at this point. Second, you need to know what they have to sell. You can waste a lot of time trying to get services for which your child may not even be eligible.

Finding Services in Your Area

Begin by asking, "Where are the services for children with autism in my area?" In public education there are often special education regions or districts that cross school district boundaries to serve all special needs children with one type of educational handicap—of which autism is one. What service area are you in? What are these areas called where you live? Are you acquainted with *all* the alternatives within this area? If you live close to a border of a special education service area, what are the rules governing interdistrict transfers? There is usually a central special education office you can call to get this information. Also be aware, as we will discuss later, that not all children diagnosed with autism will need a class designed for children with autism. You should have an assessment that describes what your child needs (as discussed in Chapter 2).

Even nonpublic agencies, especially the ones that offer home-based services, don't go everywhere. Most of the agencies offering ABA/DTT services depend on a workforce of twenty-something-year-old recent college grads. This means if you're near a city or a college campus, they may all live around there—or wherever the rent is not exorbitant. For the purposes of their training, many will live near wherever the "mother ship" for their agency is. The farther you live from such a center, the harder it may be to get services or to interest an agency in taking your child on—if they will have to find and train local tutors from scratch. That is, however, doable, and the best alternative for many families.

Aging Out of Services

Because of the structure of public funding for special education for autism, there is often a shift in service provision at a child's third birthday. Increasingly, schools are forming collaborations with public agencies charged with providing Early Start or Zero to Three services to make the transition to ongoing school service at the third birthday transparent for families. That, however, is still the exception rather than the rule.

You will need to understand how this age three transition works in your area so you are not caught by a surprise exit from services as your child reaches her third birthday. Some parents who hope for services from nonpublic agencies try to hurry and get into such services just under the three-year-old wire. Sometimes this helps because it does allow service to start earlier—which on the whole is an important goal to reach. However, if the school has equally appropriate services beginning at age three (which might also include home-based programming), it may be worthwhile to see if some version of those services can be initiated as soon as you are ready to go ahead with treatment. It's hard enough to learn how to be your child's wraparound therapist. Spending time instead on endless IEP meetings, mediations, and hearings that may or may not let you keep nonpublic services is a decision that must always be weighed carefully (as will be discussed in Chapters 9 and 10).

For some children, the public education agencies have undertaken hybrid, collaborative plans wherein three-, four-, and five-year-olds with autism receive half-day public special education preschool programs and half-day home-based programming—often a good bridge to full-time school programming by the start of first grade.

A Great Program, but Great for My Child?

All parents who are out looking for programs for their child with autism have in mind one or two great programs they wish their child could attend. This is the great program that everyone wants but that no one can get into. Half the time it's not in your state—and it is not in a place where you might hope to be gainfully employed in your chosen line of work. I think of this as the pot-o'-gold program at the end of the rainbow (and I don't mean Hawaii—even though there's a rainbow on every license plate). When parents I see in California start telling me about how they've heard there are fabulous programs in North Carolina or New Jersey, I agree: wonderful programs. I know which ones they mean, and they are wonderful. It doesn't mean that they are a good fit for a particular child or that very comparable services are not available much closer to where the family already lives. Mortgaging the farm or the family's future does not guarantee a better result. Probably worse after you add in all the new stressors.

The whole beauty of the IEP is that it should be just that—an *individualized* education program. If you custom-make a suit, there's no reason it shouldn't fit like an Armani if you use good materials and attend to the details. It helps to start with good raw materials, *but know the best tailor is you.*

Caveat Emptor: Making a Smart Purchase

You are the consumer. What you need to "buy" is help for your child. When you read an issue of *Consumer Reports* in search of a new car or a new refrigerator, there is always this matrix of brands by features. The little cells in the matrix are filled with white holes, black holes, and ones that are partly black and partly white. On some level we all want as many white holes (the highest rating) possible. However, the car or fridge might have features you're not interested in purchasing. In that case, those circles will weigh less in your decision.

The most important part here is that you are the consumer. *You* are going to be the one to use the product you purchase. It needs to fit your bill. Specifically, as a parent of a child with autism, you really, really need to be able to collaborate with the people who are helping your child to prioritize what you need. This doesn't mean you sit there and they tell you what to do. (That would be like someone else deciding whether you needed a fridge with a water dispenser more than a fridge that holds gallon jugs.) But it also doesn't mean you tell them what to do—because the fridge salesperson (hopefully) knows more about fridges than you do. Going back to your child with autism, being a good consumer means acknowledging that you and the providers each bring a different sort of expertise to the table and together can create a whole life of learning experiences for your child.

Whatever the treatment providers are providing you, it's a product you're purchasing not just for your child but for yourself as well. Can you reach out to the service providers on behalf of your child? (Your child needs you to be able to do this.) What will be your opportunities to see what they do? How will you get supported to carry on with similar goals at home and in the community? Can you live with the approach they take? If it differs from your family culture or values, can you ask for help to understand better what they feel needs to be done? What you are looking for is a team you can join.

PART III

Putting It Together

MATCHING YOUR CHILD'S
LEARNING NEEDS WITH
THE TREATMENTS THAT CAN HELP

You know your child's diagnosis. You've learned what services are available to you. Which do you choose? You've heard that earlier is better. You already feel like you should have known what was going on sooner and gotten treatment started six months ago. Does that mean that you should take the first program that has an opening? You've also heard that intensity is important. Does that mean you should take the program that offers the most hours?

What you will learn in the next three chapters is how to move forward with the information you have from your diagnostic assessments, from cruising the Internet, and from identifying the therapists, schools, and public service agencies that are there to help families with autistic children. How do you take the information you have and use it to understand which services will be the best fit for your child's learning strengths and weaknesses?

You are already an expert on your child from living with him and from trying all the things that naturally occurred to you to do to help him. How do you merge your expertise with the assessment information and fit it to the services that are out there?

Beyond diagnostic assessment, you will need a finer understanding of your child's specific learning strengths and weaknesses. You will need to know which programs and approaches help which kinds of children most.

What about the *content*, the *curriculum* of the programs that you're considering? More hours of a program that doesn't address your child's specific learning problems are not going to be as good as choosing one that can. It's not a matter of what you can get first or what can give you the most hours of service. It's about tailoring any good program to fit your child's individual strengths and weaknesses.

In the next three chapters, I'll cover three closely related topics:

Chapter 6 will teach you how to scrutinize your child's learning style. I'll talk about how your child's weak areas can be classified as different autism-specific learning disabilities (ALDs). The ALD concept provides a template for converting the checklist of your child's specific autism symptoms into a checklist of his autism-specific learning weaknesses and autism-specific relative learning strengths. I will also talk about autistic learning styles (ALSs), which are ways of taking relative strengths or seemingly odd talents (like feats of memory or an ability to know which buttons to press) and putting them into service as tools for learning things your child needs to learn—like learning how to talk.

Then, in Chapter 7, once you are armed with your new understanding of your child's specific learning strengths and weaknesses, I'll discuss the best aspects of each of the main approaches to autism treatment. I'll give you a travelogue through the alphabet of autism treatment buzzwords you'll have encountered—like DTT, PRT, TEACCH, DIR, RDI, and others. To get some assurance that your child's learning needs are going to be addressed by a treatment you're considering, I'll show you how to cross-tabulate your child's ALDs by the strengths of each of these treatment approaches. This will let you see what you can expect your child to get from a particular treatment approach, as well as what might not be fully addressed and require some additional services to cover all your need treatment bases.

Then in Chapter 8, we'll look at additional strategies that target specific problems in specific areas of development like motivation, peer relationships, and developing language understanding and an ability to talk. Throughout Part III I'll talk about where you as the parent fit into treatment. In Chapter 8, I'll talk about "the wraparound parent"—how you can cement formal learning experiences by making what the child learns in school into "news he can use" in navigating his everyday needs.

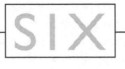

SIX

Learning Deficits, Learning Styles

WHAT DOES *YOUR* CHILD NEED?

If you want to have an idea of the challenges your child will face as he begins to participate in any treatment program that you select for him, imagine the following: Let's start simple. If I asked you what it was like to be deaf, you could watch TV for an hour with the sound off. See how much you "get." If I asked you to imagine being blind, you could put on a blindfold. (Recently on National Public Radio there was a story about a restaurant somewhere in Scandinavia run by the blind partly as a self-help project, partly to increase awareness of blindness. You come into the restaurant and it is pitch black. The maître d' as well as all wait staff are blind. You are led to your table. You listen to the menu, you order, and then you grope around for utensils and the location of the food on your plate. Pretty tough . . .)

Now let's make this exercise more difficult: Image you are autistic. Maybe the language you hear rushes by, with only a few words you really know popping up. You focus on those and then try to figure out the rest from what's going on around you. You repeat the part you understood, trying to link it to something else. You like things to be routine and predictable—because then, at least, you have a pretty good idea of what's going to happen next even if you can't understand what's being said or what is meant by the words you hear and can repeat. When things you expect to happen don't, you feel really aggravated and maybe lash out at the person who violated your expectations. When other kids are around, you start to freak out, run away or at least turn away, and block them out. They are completely unpredictable. Maybe some talking or sounds are too loud, so you hum or moan or cover your ears to drown out the senseless noise. Just like sounds being too loud sometimes, things that touch you might feel "too loud," the volume turned up too high. Certain movements might make you feel the volume is turned up too high too. Other sounds, tactile sensations, or rhythmic movement you crave and want to find a way to amplify.

What's Inside the World of the Autistic Child?

We don't exactly know all the distortions that make unexpected impressions and create the very different internal world of the child with autism. We do know that there are systematic alterations in the way the child perceives information—through hearing, how things are looked at, responses to touch, spatial orientation and equilibrium, and so on. Then there are alterations in the speed at which information can move through the brain, the "signal" (sight, sound, touch—whatever) degrading, becoming less fully representative of the initial perception as processing takes longer and longer. Then a faulty signal, once processed, might not get stored as something meaningful in the intended way. If the input to the child (the signal) degrades, maybe only part is stored (like the sound of the word but not its meaning). If information doesn't fully get to where it should be going or is only partly stored, the downstream snippets, odds and ends, bits and pieces are fragmentary, and retrieval and expression can't possibly be spot on.

The best we can do is to make up a list of all the inputs that can go astray—that are received to weakly, too strongly, or too slowly. We need to do this for every sense—hearing, vision, the senses of taste and touch, the senses of movement and pressure. We need to know what the autistic child pays too little attention to and too much attention to. As we begin to think of an individual child with autism in this way, we start to see how she can be helped to compensate for what is weakest by using the capacities that are developing more as expected.

This chapter defines various *autism-specific learning disabilities* (ALDs) to help you become aware of which ones are most at issue for your child. By the end of the chapter, you'll have a better sense of your child's ALD *profile*, which will help you begin to see where her learning deficits and styles dovetail with the offerings of the main treatment approaches for autism, the subject of Chapter 7. Knowing as specifically as possible where there's a fit between what your child needs and what a treatment provides is the surest route to the best help for your child with minimal tangents and detours.

Autism as a Compilation of ALDs

An ALD is something that causes a child with an autism spectrum disorder to learn something differently from the way others his age do. We know children with autism learn to talk differently. They learn social skills differently. They learn to play with toys differently from others their age. These differences are all domains of disparate kinds of ALDs. When you understand these, you'll have a better idea of what makes your child with autism tick.

By developing a fuller understanding of how your child can and can't learn, you'll have identified where you and the rest of your child's treatment team can begin to make a difference with strategies for using the stronger abilities to boost the weaker ones. You can do this *regardless* of the diagnostic label he's received—if some of your child's learning differences are the same ones that are common to children with autism.

If you emerged from your child's diagnostic assessment with no clear answer about why one treatment might be better than another, you may feel condemned to a sort of limbo—not knowing which road heads most directly to help for your child, despite the fact that you know (and the experts agree) that there is indeed something awry with your child's development. Understanding that there is no single symptom of autism that occurs just in children with autism or an autism spectrum disorder, as explained in Chapters 1 and 3, can help you see that thinking in terms of ALDs will clear a road to the most tailored treatment even if your child really doesn't meet enough criteria to be called autistic or PDD. Many individual symptoms of autism spectrum disorders occur just as commonly in children with severe language delays or disorders or in children with mental retardation.

Various techniques have been developed to treat specific ALDs in children with autism but work comparably well for these other children. A good example is the picture communication systems (discussed in detail in Chapter 8) developed for autism. A method like the Picture Exchange Communication System (PECS) was devised using broad-based behavior modification techniques that can help non-autistic kids too. That's because PECS, while designed to acknowledge that autistic children are often much stronger at visual than verbal recognition, may be just as suitable for other children who are specifically and significantly delayed in beginning to talk, *if* they too are stronger visually than verbally—though they may play and interact socially much better than a child with autism. The system doesn't target just kids who have autistic social deficits.

So, we could say that these significantly language-delayed children (as well as the children with autism) have one *kind* of autistic learning disability. They resemble children with autism with respect to their markedly poor verbal over visual recognition of objects and with respect to their *autistic learning style* (ALS) in that they readily compensate when pictures are closely paired with words. Some children can have one or more ALDs or ALSs—but not necessarily have enough other signs of autism to be diagnosed autistic or even PDD. This doesn't mean they won't benefit from many of the treatments designed for autism; there is every reason to expect they can.

Here's another example: Most young autistic children will not repeat a behavior just because it has been socially praised. The same is often true for children with moderate to severe mental retardation. So, if we want to condition the child to repeat a desirable behavior when praised by a teacher or Mom or Dad, we have to use another, stronger *primary* reinforcer, such as food and sensory rewards. Pairing primary reinforcers with social reinforcers in this way can be said to address an autistic learning disability—a lack of response to social praise—in both children with autism and children with mental retardation.

Now, let's translate this concept of autism-specific learning disability into the concept of autistic learning *style*. If the child must learn to respond to social praise through conditioning, rather than responding to praise innately, we can say that the child has an autistic learning style with respect to how he has had to learn response to social praise.

The bottom line is that, if your child has an autistic learning style in any of the areas discussed in the rest of this chapter, she stands to benefit from teaching strategies designed for that style, *irrespective of diagnosis*. In fact, in my own experience, many children with some ALDs or some ALSs (who don't meet the full medical criteria for autism) may get "educationally" diagnosed as autistic because parents find that programs for children with autism spectrum disorders are a better fit than other categories of special education service they encounter.

Constructing Your Child's Learning Profile

ALDs can be viewed as falling into three categories: social deficits, communication deficits, and deficits in organizing information. I'll describe each of these in turn. As you read, there will be checklists to help you keep track of which you feel are areas of concern for your child.

Which *Social* ALDs Does Your Child Have?

Let's start with how the social deficits we associate with autism affect learning. We can refer to these as "social ALDs." Central to autism is the child's lack of social and emotional reciprocity: The child often has a lack of desire to please others. The child often does not respond to social praise until explicitly conditioned to have that response, as just described. This apparent lack of interest in earning the approval of others often links up with an apparent lack of concern about the effect the child's own actions may have on others. The upshot is that the child's motivations are often geared toward pleasing himself foremost, with relatively less concern for others' goals if they conflict with his own.

Okay, you knew all this. But what does it mean for the child's ability to learn? It means that the child with autism is "DC" in an "AC" world. His motivational system, his little engine that propels him further, is in reverse. The child with autism is instrumental. He will approach others not just expecting them to drop everything and pay attention to him but for the specific reason that he needs something he can't get for himself. Think what that means: Every time a ten-month-old points at something and says "Dat!" we parents can't do enough to make "Dat" into a lesson. If the child points out a window, Dad might typically carry the child to the window, say "What do you *see*?" and then give a rhetorical answer: "Oh, you *see* Mommy coming!" That's a whole lot of lessons for a ten-month-old:

1. Pointing is associated with someone else seeing what you see.
2. Pointing gets you moved in the direction in which you point.
3. That word *see* has to do with what you pay attention to.
4. "Mommy" (who, of course, is Mommy) is what I see.

The child with autism lacks the basic understanding that you see what I see when we both look at it. Sometimes this is referred to as the child lacking a theory of mind. The child's ability to "theorize" that others are seeing and feeling what he sees and feels is sometimes also called *intersubjectivity.* Another way to explain this is simply to say that from about the age of ten months on, the typically developing child can tell when he and a parent are on the same page—and he'll work hard to have that happen. The young child intuitively understands that when the two of you are on the same page, you can "read" that page to him, explain all about it, and enhance his own feelings of excitement (or assuage feelings of anxiety) through your reactions and explanations.

Nobody teaches children to do this; it's an innately arising capacity. But it needs to be taught to children with autism if they are to access all the information on any "page." An absence of this theory of mind (or being on the same page) has profound implications for learning: By the time the child is twenty months old, think about how many opportunities for lessons have been missed!

So not being able to understand that others can see what you can see is an autistic learning disability. This means *lack of theory of mind*—not just lack of social and emotional reciprocity or lack of interest in others or lack of concern about the effects of one's actions on others—*is the core ALD.* When thinking of treatment needs, thinking about treating the core problem of same-pageness is where it is at and will imbue what you need to think about as you look toward teaching social skills, play skills, and language.

What else goes with this? The child with autism is not just out there looking for an excuse to redirect attention to himself. The typical two-year-old will repeat any silly little thing just to get you to look at him. He craves information input. The child with autism does not usually crave information input from people. But he should, because it drives learning opportunities; it drives opportunities to practice and sustain back-and-forth social interaction. So a low desire for social input is another dimension of social ALD. This low drive can be thought of as connected to the difficulties with theory of mind just discussed. The child just does not yet see why having fun can be even more fun if someone else who is important in his life is having fun with him.

This translates into what happens when the child goes to pre-school. The teacher says she wants all the children who are ready for a story to take their mat to circle, sit criss-cross, and raise their hand when they are quiet and have their listening ears on. On the first day of school, an aide may help motor a new child through this routine, but counts on his picking it up quickly. Why? Because everyone else is do-ing it. As the teacher calls out names of who has "ready listening ears," others hurry up and raise a hand—because each child wants to hear the teacher call *his* name and praise *his* listening readiness. If a pre-school teacher couldn't depend on this uniform desire to please her, and on the desire to want to do what others in the peer group want to, teaching every preschool class would be like herding cats. This brings us to another aspect of social ALD—a lack of desire to do like and be like peers. It's pretty obvious how this limits learning in a group-based setting.

Let's skip ahead to thinking about treatment for a minute: If a child with autism is totally and absolutely uninterested and unable to learn or be motivated by peers, does teaching him in a group help? In-stead, what about formally teaching some imitation skills one to one and then reevaluating the appropriateness of group-based teaching where imitation of others can really teach and motivate the develop-ment of new skills? In the next chapter, you will begin to see how pro-grams for autism fit these ALDs. ABA/DTT programs, for example, teach one to one and teach formal imitation skills to children who lack any concept of imitating. If they also lack a response to social praise, they teach that too. So, when there's no imitation and no response to social praise, DTT makes a lot of sense. What is also true is that as a child starts to gain these skills, he has gained some of the prerequisites for being able to learn in a group.

Following are checklists to help you examine the extent to which your child has social ALDs related to the capacity to understand the self in relation to others. You can answer yes or no but might also want to keep track of whether this is:

- 1—a very marked problem,
- 2—definitely an issue, or
- 3—an issue, but not really a problem.

Social ALDs Related to Social Understanding

Does your child need help becoming more AWARE OF OTHERS?   Yes?

Acts as if in own little world.	
Foremost motivation is usually to please self.	
More readily learns things that result in meeting own needs.	
Fails to notice certain things that others this age usually notice.	
May behave as if unaware that caregivers are in the same room.	
Seems to lack a desire to do things just to please others.	

For some children with autism, the inability to respond to emotions in others limits how their behavior can be modulated by parents and teachers. Many parents have "tested" this in their children by pretending to cry or be seriously hurt to see if their child would notice or respond. One mother told me she even lay on the floor for several minutes, pretending to be dead, to see if her two-and-a-half-year-old son would notice. It's pretty conspicuous when a young child doesn't respond to such a ploy. What it means for learning is pretty conspicuous too. A teacher depends on keeping things moving smoothly by being able to call a child's name and just give her a look to indicate whether what the teacher sees is what she's expecting. The child who does not, or cannot, receive such signals is not helping herself help the teacher to teach her best. Does the child know when her teacher (or her mom) really means business? Isn't it sad that just a smile or a nod for a job well done might not have the intended reinforcing effect? Identifying such deficits as particular holes in a child's information processing—yet another dimension of social ALD—puts something else on the list that must be taught if the child is going to be able to learn more like others his age.

Does your child have difficulty reading and responding to EMOTIONS? Yes?

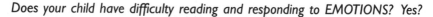

Doesn't modify actions if someone else gets sad/pretends sadness.	
Doesn't look around to see who notices when he/she cries.	
Doesn't clearly look pleased when verbally praised (like "Great job!").	
Can't be counted on to repeat an action that's been verbally praised.	
Apparent lack of awareness about the effect of his behavior on others.	

Imitation is a major way that the typically developing toddler learns. It is said that imitation is the sincerest form of flattery, and so it's not surprising that the first peer relationships are partly built on imitation. Imitation of an action or an activity is like a small video clip from someone else's library that a child takes into his own video library. Once it's there, the child can use it to write scripts for fresh takes on the clip he has. When a four-year-old sees another boy grinding a handle that makes a dump truck dump, he "videos" it, later literally replaying it. Then he can literally play with variations on the theme. When the capacity for imitation is absent or only very selectively present, it too constitutes another ALD.

Imitation can be seen as driven by an innate desire to "do like" and "be like" others. A lack of imitation skills is just one manifestation of the lack of an innate drive to affiliate with others. The other main aspect of the desire to do like and be like others is the desire for peer relationships: Put two nine-month-olds who've never met on the floor with a bunch of toys and see what they do: They spot each other right away, one crawls to the other, maybe grasps a fist full of hair and makes the other cry, but each finds the other the most novel thing around. We don't teach children this—it just happens. This is what leads to observation of the other; then parallel imitative play of the other; and, finally, reciprocal play. If you're not interested in peers, you're not going to be interested in observing, imitating, and joining them. This is yet another form of ALD.

Does your child have a hard time learning new things by IMITATING? Yes?

Isn't interested in trying to do new things just to earn approval of others.	
Doesn't seem to be motivated to copy actions or attitudes of others.	
Doesn't readily learn by being shown; must figure it out on his/her own.	
Doesn't copy others just to be "cool" or appear more grown up.	
Low level of interest in peers.	
Acts as though other children (aside from siblings) are not even there.	
Shows more interest in younger children than those his own age.	
Shows more interest in older children than those his own age.	
No interest in participating in group games with other children the same age.	

Which ALDs Related to *Communication* Does Your Child Have?

In addition to all the specifically social deficits that characterize autism and that can influence the capacity to learn, be motivated, and interact socially, there are specific ALDs related to communication. Communication is really an umbrella term for formal and informal systems people have of sending feelings and thoughts back and forth. There are two main components of communication: The first to develop is "nonverbal" communication or what is more commonly referred to as "body language." The second to develop is spoken language. Both of these areas of development can be affected in children with autism. Difficulties in these areas also have immeasurable effects on how a child gets information and constructs an understanding of his world.

Body language is really every baby's first language. When development goes as planned, we speak first with our eyes, then our mouths (smiles and frowns), and later with our whole bodies. Body language is often remarkably absent from the child with an autism spectrum disorder. Even in adults who have plenty of words, facial expression and body language provide punctuation and timbre. (Ever watch an Italian drive and talk on a cell phone at the same time?)

Adults with Asperger syndrome are often remarkably still. I can think of one video I have of an adult with Asperger syndrome that I once fast-forwarded to find a specific part. As I watched the tape go forward, I realized only the mouth, not the body, was moving. It was hard to follow his narrative; and part of the reason was his poor ability to understand his listener's perspective—but part was his failure to pause, punctuate, and modulate with his face and body. One perspective is that this channel of communication is missing because it isn't a channel to which an individual with autism subscribes.

Back to the classroom. The teacher teaches with her words, but she also teaches with her face, her hands, her tone of voice. If she happens to point to a picture in a book or a word on the blackboard, being able to follow a point is a handy skill. It's not even taught in preschool. A preschool teacher, and everyone up the line, takes point following as a given, just as they assume pupils will respond to a stern prohibiting voice, a shake of the head "no," or a wave to "come here" or "go there." What happens when the child with autism does not get these signals? Typically, he's seen as either defiant or dumb.

What we actually have, though, is another area of autism-specific learning disability. Much information, especially social information, is conveyed with the face, tone of voice, and gesture. Until the child can be helped to understand the nonverbal signals, she's going to miss a whole lot of what's being communicated. This is an especially inopportune disability if you are also missing some of the signals on the other main communication channel—spoken language.

Body Language and Nonverbal Communication

Difficulty READING BODY LANGUAGE?

	Yes?
Doesn't look to the place where something is pointed out.	
Doesn't stop an action when you shake your head "no."	
Doesn't stop an action when just receiving a stern look.	
Doesn't stop an action when you shake your head "no" *and* look stern.	
A strict, serious tone of voice saying "No!" doesn't inhibit action.	
Unaware that a nod "yes" or a smile means that what s/he's doing is okay.	

Difficulty SHOWING what s/he means WITH BODY LANGUAGE?

	Yes?
Doesn't point with an index finger at things desired.	
Doesn't point at something and then look to see if you've seen it too.	
Doesn't look back after seeing something to see if you've seen it too.	
Doesn't make sure you're looking before communicating with you.	
Doesn't smile in response when someone else smiles at him or her.	
Doesn't look worried if someone on TV cries, is sad, or is hurt.	
Doesn't look happy if others act happy, like after a happy ending on TV.	
Waves bye-bye only when s/he wants to leave, is leaving, or afterward.	
You can't clearly read the emotion of shame on the child's face.	
You can't clearly read the emotion of guilt on the child's face.	
You can't clearly see when the child feels proud.	

Talking

Learning to talk for the purposes of sharing thoughts and feelings with someone else is a universal problem for children with autism spectrum disorders. However, there are many variations on this theme: Some children with autism—perhaps 20–30%—never learn to verbalize. Almost all of these children are among those autistic children who also have some degree of mental retardation. But most of these children develop a very specific autistic leading style, which is that they will hand-lead or push adults (or an adult's hand) toward what they want. They don't throw Dad's hand at the refrigerator door just to be cute, but rather in a down-to-business, unmistakably urgent way. It's instrumental communication—literally using another as an instrument— and it often works quite well for the child. What does this tell us? One thing is that the child with autism seems indeed to be "thinking in pictures," as well-known author Temple Grandin described her own autistic learning style.* The child understands that the hand must go to the fridge door before the door opens—so he makes it go. His way of talking about what he wants is not with words, not with a point, but with literally seeing it happen. These are clues—that helping the child visualize what will happen plays to his autistic learning style. In the next section as we talk about treatment approaches, we'll cover TEACCH, an approach that makes significant use of picture schedules, visual schedules, and visual icons of all sorts. This is another foreshadowing of how a list of a child's specific ALDs (and ALSs) can be a guide to selecting a program that is tailored to how a particular child learns.

There are other kinds of communicative ALDs that affect how a child with autism communicates. There are two levels of these. More severely affected children, and often younger children, have significant auditory processing problems. The sound just moves too fast—like when you go to Mexico on holiday and haven't tried to speak Spanish since Spanish II in high school. Do you get 25%? Probably not. If you catch a noun or two in a couple of sentences, you're doing great. You probably do better at catching *cerveza* if the waiter is pointing to a bottle of beer on the menu as he says it. This is because the word is coming at you already decoded. You'll likely remember it better under those

---

*Temple Grandin is a woman with very-high-functioning autism who has written a number of memoirs about what it is like for her to try to make sense of the world; one is called *Thinking in Pictures*.

circumstances too—word and picture paired together. So will your child with autism. Think about a typically developing one- to two-year-old. Do they prefer picture stories or ones with just words? They are captivated by the pictures, as well as any gestures or changes in voice you use to amplify meaning. The autistic child has to rely more on pictures, because those gesture and tone-of-voice channels may not be part of his channel subscription.

Problems UNDERSTANDING LANGUAGE the ways others do?	Yes?
Difficult to tell if child is not understanding words or just not complying.	
Seems that child understands only when he wants to understand.	
Understands names of things (nouns) better than action words (verbs).	
May figure out what is meant by nouns plus what he sees happening.	

Problems USING LANGUAGE the way others do? (Verbal children)	Yes?
Uses words only when useful to get immediate needs met.	
Doesn't use words just to comment on interesting things.	
Doesn't chat or converse even with babbling.	
Echoes some of your speech as if to show he's with the conversation.	

Does Your Child Have ALDs Related to *Organizing Information*?

A final area where ALDs occur is in distortions in organizing incoming information. There are three dimensions to these ALDs:

　1. *Playing with things the same way over and over,* with no apparent interest in trying to use toys in new ways. This includes problems in using toys to develop a story line—like having the dolls do something *after* they eat or having the train go somewhere rather than just around the track without any stops. There is a close link between language and play, and this can be due, at least in part, to a lack of words to create a script for more elaborate play. This area of difficulty also relates back to one of the areas of social ALDs we discussed, a lack of drive to imitate—in this case, to re-create things your child is seeing and experiencing personally.

2. *Difficulty with responding to new things.* While most young children prefer a new toy, autistic children can be much more comfortable with the familiar. To some extent, this can be understood as a problem with how fast their little brain modems can take in new information—with some kinds of incoming data being harder to put through than others. The important thing here, though, is that eschewing things that are new and novel in favor of things that are old and familiar limits the numbers and variety of learning experiences the child will tend to seek out on his own.

3. *An impaired ability to reconstruct a semblance of his world through play.* This type of autistic learning disability can be associated with the language difficulties frequently seen in children with autism. Trouble comprehending action words, adjectives, and adverbs (compared to object labels—nouns) can create gaping holes in what your child understands from what is being said to him as you try to play with him and give him new ideas of what to do with his toys. Developmentally, reenacting things experienced in play usually depends to a great extent on how much language a child understands. A child who has no action words is going to demonstrate less action and less narration during play. If the child's vocabulary does not yet include adjectives (*big* car wreck) or adverbs (crashing *loudly*), you are not as likely to see those actions in her play. This defines for us another individual area of autism-specific learning disability to treat—linking language and play.

Does your child PLAY with toys differently from others his/her age? Yes?	
Toy play is mainly one action per toy—like car crashes, plane flies.	
Plays with toys, but without acting out a scene or story.	
Sets up a tableau of toys, but is then finished; no action.	
Doesn't copy actions of people with dolls, figures, or animals.	
Doesn't copy actions of videos with dolls, figures, or animals.	
Doesn't use sounds to narrate play, like crashing, or animal noises.	
Doesn't use words to narrate play.	

Signal-to-Noise Ratio Problems

Some scientists have theorized that much of what goes wrong with autism is a signal-to-noise ratio problem, meaning that autistic children have great difficulty filtering relevant signals from noise. (And neuroimaging has shown that there are some phenomena in the brain that look like this is happening.) In behavioral terms, we're talking about what is technically called *stimulus overselectivity*, meaning that your child pays too much attention to some things and too little to others. Think of the child who gets overexcited when she sees something spinning but doesn't seem to hear you calling her name. Sometimes atypical and interfering responses to sensory things disrupt the functioning you'd expect from a typical child. Maybe your child gags at the sight of a food that is not one of her accepted three foods or struggles each time you put long pants on her—even in a Minnesota winter.

On the other hand, there are children with autism who are unusually reinforced by a particular sensory sensation, like movement. If you view this "favoritism" as an ALS, you can use it to teach something important. Picture your child on a swing, with you in front of him, catching his feet with each swing, letting go only when he catches your eye. In this way, you make lemonade from lemons: Instead of just letting your child swing in an endlessly demanded, repetitive, unelaborated pattern, you've used its strong positive value to your son to get him to do something he might not otherwise do: make eye contact. Similarly, you can view—and capitalize on—your child's favoring other sensory things, like rubbing, squishing, bouncing, or certain sounds, to teach something that an ALD may seem to put out of his reach.

Does your child overreact or underreact to some SENSORY STIMULI? Yes?

Seems actually not to hear (not just ignore) some sounds/speech.	
Seems oversensitive to some sounds as too loud.	
Has very positive response to movement—like swinging or bouncing.	
Has very negative response to tactile irritations—like shirt labels, tight sleeves.	
Puts nonfood items in mouth, as if this aids in learning about them.	
Is picky about textures in mouth and what is chewed or swallowed.	

When There's Not Much Curiosity

One way we catch autism early is through parent reports that the child seems to concentrate incredibly well on certain things while ignoring other things. This can turn out to be the autistic child with very little curiosity. Why is curiosity so important? Young children have been described by developmental psychologists as little scientists, doing the same and similar things over and over as a way to learn from their own actions. If you don't explore, you don't learn. I always think of times when a new three-year-old child comes to my clinic for assessment—along with an eighteen-month-old sibling about whom parents have no concerns. There are lots of toys. In the first hour, the eighteen-month-old may play with twenty or thirty of them, then go back to a couple he liked the best. His older brother, however, may have come in, spied the bead roller coaster, and after a half hour have checked out nothing else. The eighteen-month-old has had twenty to thirty times as many learning experiences in just that half hour as his autistic brother has had. What has this meant over the three years of the older child's life? Lack of exploratory drive can therefore be characterized as an aspect of autism-specific learning disability.

In the next chapter, as we discuss treatment approaches, you can keep in mind those treatments that feed the child information even if he doesn't seek it. You can see how such treatments will be a particularly good fit with the type of autistic child for whom highly repetitive, nonexploratory behavior is a problem.

Does your child seem to value REPETITION and AVOID NOVELTY?   Yes?

Prefers old familiar toys to new toys.	
Initially fearful of something he now loves (for example, vacuum, carousel).	
Once something is done one way, it's always done the same way.	
Has odd little nonfunctional rituals—like drinking from only one cup.	
Prefers certain toys, but *not* for main use (for example, just to spin, make noises).	
Very focused in play with one thing, but showing good concentration.	
Won't do something just because it's new or because it's there.	
Difficult to find motivators.	

Moving On

This chapter has demonstrated how you can build on what you learned about your child from the diagnostic assessment to select treatment designed specifically for him or her. It's important to build an understanding of how your child may be encountering some autism-specific barriers to learning, which I have called ALDs, or autism-specific learning disabilities. By looking closely at what a child does do, rather than just what is expected and is not happening, we can begin to realize how the ALDs have reshaped the child's ability to learn. Our job is to put effort into identifying how and why the child relates like he does, talks like he does, and plays with toys like he does—to get a toehold on how teaching can improve on and expand these natural ways the child is already starting to do things. This is what I have sometimes referred to as ALSs, or autistic learning styles.

As you think about these ALDs and ALSs for your child, you can also think back to what you've learned from diagnostic assessments. Does the information gibe with what you've been told about relative language weaknesses or sensory difficulties? Think about how having had those identified for you can be used to recast that information as your child's profile of ALDs and ALSs. This will be your guide as you begin to imagine how your child might benefit from different treatment approaches you can consider.

In the next chapter, the second step in this process, I will guide you through the different main approaches to treating autism. Each of these approaches offers a number of advantages with respect to different learning disabilities. But, to cut to the chase, you'll learn that no one approach does everything for everyone. You need to learn the strengths of each approach and make sure you put together a program that covers all the specific learning needs of your child. We will do this by outlining the best points of each approach and then cross-tabulating each approach with the list of ALDs you've developed in this chapter.

SEVEN

Core Treatments
for Autism

WHICH INTERVENTIONS
WILL MEET YOUR CHILD'S NEEDS?

Chapter 6 explained how each child with an autism spectrum disorder has a particular profile of autism-specific learning disabilities (ALDs) and that these profiles differ—sometimes just somewhat and sometimes markedly—from child to child. Children on the autism spectrum also have autistic learning styles (ALSs)—characteristic ways that many of them compensate for relative weaknesses using relatively stronger abilities. You now know that you can come to understand your child's learning styles (ALSs) by looking closely at how he solves problems differently from other children the same age—such as relying on visual cues to know whether something he wants will happen or hand-leading you to the fridge, as if running a little instructional video on the steps needed to see what's inside.

Paying attention to where your child's learning weaknesses are, what his strengths are, and how the strengths can help compensate for the weaknesses lays the foundation for putting together a treatment plan by telling you what *your* child needs. Now you need to frame out the building, becoming familiar with the main comprehensive treatment approaches for autism—especially the key strengths of each. Once you know what your child needs and what the main treatment approaches have to offer, you can start to build the structure: to see where the best fit lies and select an approach that plays to his strengths.

As you'll see, you have lots of options, not only among the comprehensive treatment approaches covered in this chapter but also strategies from a long list of "à la carte" extras that we'll go over in the following chapter. To go back to the house-building analogy, these "extras" are your doors and windows. As general contractor, you know your house will have a floor and walls, but there will also be decisions to make about what kind of flooring—like carpet or hardwood. These are the finer details, analogous to choosing one teacher over another. It can be helpful to think of the relative importance of these design decisions, realizing that having a floor at all is more important than opting for one carpet over another—though of course it's always nice to have a choice.

While this may seem complicated at first, it really isn't: It just means that a treatment plan can and should be crafted to address your child's unique learning style profile. This is the true spirit of the term IEP, *individualized education program*—the plan for helping your child learn that you're entitled to by federal law (see Chapter 9). The plan that's best for your child is going to be the one that ensures all his ALDs are addressed fully, his strengths are recognized as tools for teaching him to get better at the things it's hardest for him to learn, and the teaching content is geared developmentally—teaching what would come next for a typically developing child.

Catching the Spirit of the IEP

- Weaknesses (autism-specific learning disabilities) are addressed by selecting specific, targeted teaching strategies.
- Strengths (autistic learning styles) are used to determine the best modalities by which the child can learn (for example, visual, motor).
- Content taught is "what comes next" during typical development.

Trying to reach this goal of having a true made-to-order program may put you in a position you haven't been in before, of requesting a custom-tailored mix of treatments rather than the standard "package" the school system may be accustomed to offering. It is completely okay to ask for what your child needs. At this point, you have assessment data to back up your request. But don't let the IEP process become an "I want" versus "They don't want to give (because I want)" adversarial situation. When this happens, the IEP process is refocused away from the child and onto the personalities of the people who should be collaborating to write the plan. So, before you go any farther on the road to getting the best treatment for your child, I'm going to ask you to remember that you are not simply on the receiving end, seeking to "get" the treatments your child needs and deserves. You are, in fact, an integral part of the treatment team yourself and need to show what you will be doing to make a plan work.

Your job is going to be twofold: First, you are the general contractor. You make sure all the services fit together by understanding how they can be complementary. Not everybody can or should work on everything that can be helpful to your child's learning: There are some things that speech and language therapists do, other things that behaviorists do, and so on. This means that in addition to being the general contractor, you are the cement subcontractor—you make it all hold together.

As we've been discussing, learning occurs during formal teaching or therapy, but also whenever your child needs, wants, or can be interested in something in her world that can be of some educational value to her. So as general contractor you need to be aware of what each other subcontractor is building, but as cement subcontractor you also need to provide wraparound opportunities whenever there is a natural chance to practice emerging skills that are just being taught or that will benefit from reinforcement in natural situations. This will cement the learning. Keep this dual role in mind as you think about the fit between your child's ALD/ALS learning profile and each of the treatments discussed in the following pages.

The Fixed-Price Meal versus Ordering à la Carte

Another good way to begin to think about the main, comprehensive treatments for autism is to think about going to a rather nice restaurant and finding that they have a very appealing fixed-price multicourse dinner listed on the left side of the menu. Really elegant, you think. For what a starter, an entrée, and a dessert might cost, you'll also get a soup, a salad, a couple of side dishes with your entrée, and a beverage to boot. Just as you've made up your mind, however, your eye drifts to the other side of the menu. They have a ribeye steak—you love ribeye. You were thinking the duck on the prix fixe would be great, but you decide to ask the waiter whether you can make a substitution. What does he say? No, of course.

This is how I regard the problem with many of the comprehensive treatments for autism: The ABA/DTT folks say they've got it all covered. You want your child to talk? We'll start with verbal imitation drills. You want your child to learn to copy other kids? No problem; we'll start with nonverbal imitation drills.

They're not wrong—but there are other methods too. What about TEACCH? Its developers tout its "cradle to grave" applicability. They're not wrong either. But are they talking about treating the same kinds of children with autism as the ABA/DTT folks? I'll give you a closer look in the following pages so you can see whether both programs seem equally suitable for your child. One program might be a better fit than others at different stages of your child's development or different ages. What about a hybrid program?

If you were rich enough, you'd tell the waiter at that fancy restaurant to bring the ribeye anyway and give the duck to a poor deserving waiter. Like a rich guy at a restaurant, you need to learn to take the best and leave the rest.

Fortunately, you don't have to be rich to get the specific services that match your child's needs because you're entitled to an individualized program by law as we will discuss fully in Chapter 9. Let's say your child is able to learn from one-to-one direct work with a speech and language pathologist but cannot yet benefit from the same work in a group. This means that taking one-to-one speech and language therapy but leaving group speech and language therapy may make sense right now. Your child may learn well in discrete trials, but also learn well when a very directive older child is with him one to one. Build that in too.

Think about what your child needs, not just what is offered. An offer of services, either from a school or from a private provider, is just that—an offer. You are your child's general contractor: Do you need or want what's offered? Do you have reason to believe the offer is too little? Too much? Not the right services? Your first step is to identify the core program—or programs, if a hybrid looks like truly the best

option—that appears likely to do the most for your child, and that's
the focus of this chapter. Then you can learn about the additional strategies (the "à la carte interventions") that will maximize your child's
learning in specific areas that are typically problematic for kids with
autism and need extra attention. These strategies, described in Chapter
8, are ones you can adopt at home and also make sure are incorporated
into your child's IEP to compose a truly comprehensive and individualized treatment program.

Always remember that a more costly program does not necessarily make the best-tailored program. The overall program that stimu-
lates and expands all the different ways and places in which your child
can learn will give you the best quality of service, and not necessarily
at the highest price.

The Main Approaches for Treating Autism

There are four main groupings for the various kinds of core programs
available to treat autism, shown in the table on this page. Some children, especially the youngest children starting treatment for the first
time, are placed in one-to-one treatments. Discrete trial training (DTT)
programs, which are sometimes referred to as ABA (applied behavior
analysis) programs, are the ones parents hear about most often: Many
children with the best outcomes have had these services, though there
are also many examples of children who do just as well with other
kinds of intensive services. (DTT is, in fact, just one set of ABA

Dimensions of Autism Treatment Programs

	Adult-led	Child-led
One-to-one treatment	Discrete trial training (ABA/DTT, aka Lovaas Therapy) Pivotal response training (PRT/incidental teaching)	Floortime (DIR) Relationship Development Interaction (RDI) Hanen
	Special education	**General education**
Classroom-based	TEACCH "Communication" classes "Noncategorical" special day classes	Inclusion/mainstreaming Resource specialist program, (RSP) support

methods—so to be extremely accurate, these terms should not be inter-changed.) DTT programs most often are one-to-one programs where the adult works from a very structured curriculum and leads the child, step by step, through a series of repeated activities until a substantial level of mastery is achieved

A simple example of an early ABA/DTT activity might be to teach your child to "stand up" and "sit down" on verbal request. At first the child might need to be physically moved through the whole sequence (called *motor prompting*) and rewarded for any degree of success along the way. As soon as a success is achieved, motor prompting is lessened, bit by bit, until the child responds independently and is rewarded just once for a complete success.

DTT can be contrasted most easily with more child-led one-to-one programs. By "child-led," I mean programs where the child's activity sets the scene. A key distinguishing element of these programs is that the child is motivated by leading the way into activity or by making choices among relatively preferred activities. Letting the child exert a preference builds in a natural reinforcement system, so there tends to be much less dependence on food and sensory rewards that aren't inherently related to the tasks at hand than there is in the early stages of many DTT programs. (A child-led teaching episode would be built on something of natural interest to the child, like sending marbles down a ramp. Over time, the adult would add ideas to the play so that sending Matchbox cars and little people down the same ramp would be just as likely to be among the child's self-initiated activities.)

One-to-one programs provide the opportunity to absolutely individualize curriculum, pacing, and content to address a child's specific learning style, developmental level, and motivational issues. However, life is not one to one, nor should teaching eternally be. At some point, learning in a group can be advantageous as peers provide vicarious observational practice of skills that your child too will be learning. A group provides incidental natural opportunities to use new words, ideas, play "scripts," and so on for your child to operate successfully under her own steam. Depending on both readiness criteria and available alternatives, most children can benefit from education in a group setting once they gain some receptive language, imitation, and control of behaviors that are incompatible with learning. A child with autism who gets to such a point can benefit from full-time or at least part-time placement in some sort of group. Depending on how different your child's level of development is from those of her age, the better fit could be either a special education classroom or a general education classroom (usually with supports at first).

Now let's take a more detailed look at each of these types of core programs with an eye to whether your child might benefit from a program that includes features of each.

Adult-Led One-to-One Focused Approaches to Treating Autism

You can read about using one-to-one behavioral modification methods to treat autism in numerous places—mainly, as I've already mentioned, about discrete trial training and how it works. These range from inspirational first-person accounts (like *Let Me Hear Your Voice*) to how-to manuals (like *A Work in Progress*) to some of the actual research (like Lovaas's 1987 publication in *Mental Retardation*) (see Resources at the end of this book). What you won't find in any of this literature, though, is a critique of the strengths and weaknesses of DTT compared to other approaches. For whom is DTT best? What about other behavioral methods like pivotal response training (PRT)? Is it better? Is it different? Do you use it instead? Do you use it together with DTT? What kinds of autism-related learning problems is it most powerful at addressing? What kinds of autism-related learning problems is it poorest at addressing?

If your child does need DTT, who pays for it? Some schools do fund DTT programs provided by nonpublic agencies headed by behaviorists with credentials like a BCBA (board-certified behavior analyst). Some schools provide DTT in school if it is recommended explicitly. Some schools have whole preschool classes for children with autism that are all DTT all the time. If this is a service that needs, at some point, to be all or part of your child's education plan, it should be made available to him. Like all services, however, its recommendation will be considered valid when it comes from an evaluator with credentials and standing with the IEP team. Since BCBAs usually have no qualifications as educators, and educators are seldom BCBAs, it can be most helpful to have the recommender of these services be someone familiar with a range of behavioral *and* educational models for treating autism. (This means that, for example, taking in a "prescription" for ABA from your pediatrician will seem quite silly and toothless to any school administrator—who can rightfully point out that the school is not a pharmacy.) In Chapter 9, we'll discuss what the law says on this topic, as knowing the legal precedents can spare you a lot of distress and increase your effectiveness as an advocate for your child.

Discrete Trial Training

At the very beginning, children with autism often have what an educator might describe as "no instructional control." You can't teach them, because they don't want to learn anything that isn't already their own idea. This limitation has a profound impact on the learning process and makes it impossible to tell which things the child *won't* learn and which she *can't* learn.

DTT is superb at establishing an "instructional contract" with a child who may seem to be in this predicament. The contract has one clause: "You need to do something to get something." On its most basic level, it boils down to something like this: You stand up as I say "Stand up!" (and I'll even help you at first), and when it's done, you get an M&M or half a Cheeto. Through the use of "shaping" (slowly changing behavior till it's the desired behavior) the child is helped to work at "Stand up!" till he can do it on his own. Each time the child is given a chance to do this, it's a "trial." Each separate chance is "discrete"—a separate opportunity. (I sometimes see people referring to this inaccurately as "discreet" trials—which would imply it was being done quietly, I suppose.) The child learns to learn with discrete trials, maybe for the first time. It's pretty wonderful to watch that little lightbulb go on for the first time.

DTT emphasizes pairing the primary reinforcers mentioned in the last chapter (food or well-regarded sensory stimulation, like a tickle) with social reinforcers like "Good job!," a high five, and the perennial favorite, "You're so smart!" Just like in Pavlov's nineteenth-century experiments with salivating dogs and a bell, eventually you can fade out the primary reinforcer and fuel the desired, new behaviors on social reinforcers that have been closely associated: A child being taught to touch a picture of Mommy when he sees it can at first be given a food treat and a cheerful "Yes!" Each time, he is coached to reach out and touch the picture. After a while, the child can have both the coaching and the food treat taken out of the picture and will look forward to that "Yes!" when he's correct. In essence, DTT assists the child to develop early cause-and-effect responding. It also develops attention to instruction by using high-value reinforcers, the highest-value reinforcers delivered most copiously when a task is newest and most difficult.

Using DTT, children can be taught the basics of imitation. Usually, young children with autism are started on so-called nonverbal imitation drills: The adult says "Do this!" (and does something like touching his own head) while a second adult prompts the child to touch his own head in the same way. "Do this!" becomes a "shutter click" on the child's internal "camera." The child preserves the event and can replicate it (immediately for the offered reinforcer or later, anytime that behavior he has learned to imitate might come in handy).

DTT can be used to teach not only nonverbal imitation but also verbal imitation: The adult, starting with some knowledge of sounds or words the child can already make, produces one sound, holding the primary reinforcer near her mouth till the child gets the idea that saying that sound—or at least at first saying *any* sound or even moving his lips slightly—is an approximation of the desired behavior that will be rewarded. Using this method, the child can be helped to produce a range of sounds and words. Verbal imitation drills can work to make indistinct articulation clearer for some children.

Importantly, DTT is adult led: First of all, the adult keeps up the pace, which is very important for the child who does not very actively seek new experiences or is highly repetitive. Second, new information is literally "on the table" every couple of minutes; every discrete trial is another opportunity to learn, consolidate knowledge, or get better. Third, the adult can choose what is learned next—structuring the order of teaching to build from basics to the more complex—as in the example given earlier of moving from lip movements to sounds to words.

Quality Assurance

So is there anything wrong with DTT? What are the possible pitfalls? For one thing, DTT is really a *method*, not a *curriculum*. The use of the discrete trials of teaching, the pairing of primary and social reinforcers, the use of prompting and prompt fading are methods that have nothing to do with the *content* of what one chooses to teach using the discrete trial method. Of course, if you buy a DTT "how-to manual," there will be curriculum. The curriculum, however, is not always what I would call "developmental"—resembling the order in which typically developing children learn things. You can use any DTT manual to better understand the discrete trial method, but I would urge you to choose your own content based on your common knowledge of what children learn "next"—such as by remembering the order in which older sibs learned things, using baby books of milestones in typically developing children, and using your observations of other kids. The reason I say this is that there *is* a reason that development progresses in a pretty fixed order (like crawling before walking): These patterns have an evolutionary basis—and correspond to proliferating structures in the brain that will be needed to support increasingly complex action and reasoning.

It can be said that typically developing children learn "horizontally," meaning they learn many examples of one thing—like "dog" to form the prototype of a dog—not "vertically" (with just one example of many things—like "dog," "cat," "horse"—before ever being exposed to a second example of each thing). Of course, very bright little autistic children with good rote memories can and do master what is taught "vertically." For example, such a child initially may be taught just three of his body parts: When single examples of those are "mastered" (recognized with about 90% accuracy), a few more will be added. Sometimes this is done to the point of absurdity, where a very clever child with autism may start with "nose" and forty body parts later be able to show you his "big toe" and his "pointer finger"— though still not yet be able to find Mommy's "nose" or the doggie's "nose" because he has had the opportunity to learn only one example for each newly "mastered" word. This is what I mean by "vertical teaching": teaching a long list that connects with nothing.

In contrast, in the language development of typically developing children, finding your own nose is quickly followed by locating Mommy's nose, your favorite nighttime lovie's nose, and Rudolph the Red-Nosed Reindeer's nose—with the big toe coming in quite a bit later. What the typically developing child does is therefore what I mean by "horizontal" learning—gaining a foundation for a concept, not simple memorization of a specific example.

An often-encountered ALS is the use of strong rote memory to compensate for all sorts of other common ALDs—like slow auditory processing, poor ability to parse words, and overall poor comprehension because of these. So, it can be a real temptation to overexploit the ALS—by just adding single examples of new words with autistic children for whom good rote auditory memory is a great compensatory strength. But we must be careful not to kid ourselves that a child really understands the word *nose* if he can find only one or two examples of it and does not yet understand that *nose* (or any noun) is actually a label for a prototype for "nose." Many people who run DTT programs will simply tell me they have not yet worked on "generalizing" an item of receptive vocabulary where the child has "mastered" his first "SD" (jargon for discriminative stimulus—that is, a single example). While what has been accomplished certainly is not *nothing*, it means almost nothing to development of functional expressive language until the child can use the word as a concept and not just a stimulus response.

This is really important, because a big complaint of parents who have used extensive DTT programs is that the child "has" a vocabulary of four to five hundred words, all carefully documented, but never uses them "spontaneously." This is why. As a parent, your really crucial job with respect to any DTT program your child may have is to leverage its benefit by providing opportunities to recognize and practice emerging vocabulary as your child naturally encounters further examples of words in his drills.

Pivotal Response Training/Incidental Teaching

DTT is Lovaas's innovation from the 1960s and 1970s. In the last thirty to forty years, you'll be glad to know, a league of next-generation researchers have laid new work on the foundations of DTT. Pivotal response training (PRT) is based on DTT and uses all its *methods*, but in ways that promote more spontaneous learning by modifying the *curriculum* that is most often used in discrete trial manualized curricula. Interestingly, the developers of PRT (like Bob and Lynn Koegel and Laura Schreibman) don't really see what they have done as being more "developmental" but rather serving motivation—which just so happens to get to be a problem when you teach children vocabulary that has no use except as a tool to obtain an external reinforcer that at any given moment they may or may not want.

In the case of PRT, behavioral and developmental goals in teaching are one and the same—teaching communication through "news you can use": Typically developing children are most interested in learning things that make life easier and more interesting—so first words include *Mommy* (who tends to respond to that word with showers of attention), *ba-ba* (like for bottle), *up* to get moved from what is currently happening to something else, and so on. Autistic children are also interested in controlling their worlds—though in a more instrumental, less social way at first. For this reason teaching them things of interest will work too. PRT has placed emphasis on giving children choices—which task to do next, to use a crayon or a pencil, to do one math problem before another—and has data to show that this improves motivation, which translates into time spent on task, quicker response times, and higher accuracy. This makes DTTs done with a PRT curriculum look more natural. While PRT developers do not emphasize teaching in developmental sequence, they emphasize teaching children to ask questions that result in interesting (reinforcing) answers.

How does this look? Here's an example: In a DTT, a child may be given a moment to use a reinforcing toy for accurately responding to "Touch nose!" In PRT, the child might be prompted to say "What is it?" when presented with a closed box, and when he responds to a prompt to say "What is it?" the box is opened, and he's told, "It's a helicopter!" and then asked: "What is it?" When the child says "helicopter," he gets to play with it. The language is immediately topical and functional, and the child is being encouraged to say "What is it?" the next time he sees a closed box he suspects holds something he likes. This difference makes PRT superior to "plain vanilla" DTT. However, PRT programs need to be very individual, very much based on a particular child's needs and interests as they come up. Much more is required of the person doing the teaching with the PRT approach than with the DTT approach. Given the simultaneous need for intensity and sustained engagement, as well as the need to use DTT as a foundation for attention and compliance so that real teaching can begin, teaching with DTT certainly has a vital place. So how do you balance the two? Here again is where you come in . . .

Where Parents Fit In

Closely aligned to the concept of PRT is the concept of incidental teaching. This is a good point to start to discuss where you as a parent fit into your child's life of learning to overcome his autism. I hope you can see from the points made in contrasting DTT and PRT that the latter is more like what naturally happens in a child's home every day. That's perfect, because every moment might be a teaching opportunity.

If your child wants something to eat, to go outside, to access a particular toy or have a favorite video on, that's a perfect time to teach. Remember that a baby just starting to talk does not say "juice," get prompted to "Say it better," and get his juice after two or three tries. A baby may start saying "num-num" for anything to eat. The parent hears "Num-num! Num-num!" and tries to guess which Num-num the baby has in mind. (The baby may help us out in a way the autistic child does not, by looking or pointing at the desired food.) The parent might say "Juice num-num?" If the baby reaches for the juice, the parent says, "Juice! You want your *juice!*" In behavioral terms, that would be called *incidental teaching.* As a parent, you can create all sorts of opportunities for incidental teaching at home and anywhere your child has a need. Although many parents realize the child with autism prizes his ability to get things for himself, they need to step in and make that just a bit more difficult each time to teach the child to stretch his abilities. This way stretching becomes rewarding, and the child wants to do more learning. How exactly is this done?

Play dumb. Lock up the videos. Take them out one at a time and ask what each one is. If the child pushes one away, say "No?" and wait for him to say "No!" before putting it away and trying with another one. Just like a parent of any child, you don't want to make this into a torture session if you know which video he wants, but give your child a really relevant experience about why having him use his words is so important to you. This very natural way of finding opportunities to practice words can be contrasted to saying "Lion King" in response to a flashcard of the *Lion King* video—but then getting a high five, not the *Lion King* video, followed by a similarly out-of-context prompt to identify *Sleeping Beauty.*

How Well Are ALDs Likely to Be Addressed?

Do you need an ABA/DTT or a PRT program? What will your child need it for? How well does it match her learning profile? Some of her autistic learning disabilities probably will be addressed, while others will not be covered. So, your child's adult-led one-to-one teaching can be just part of her overall treatment plan. The table on page 153 is a "best estimate" of how different features of such programs do or don't (or only partly) target each broad area of autistic learning disability. Note that in this table and the ones following it, I've used different formatting for the "Yes" and "Partial" table entries to make them easier to find.

Child-Led One-to-One Focused Approaches to Treating Autism

In contrast to treatments for autism that are very clearly didactic and in which the adult absolutely (DTT) or largely (PRT) decides what comes next, there are treatments where the child can lead. What do these have

How One-to-One Adult-Led (ABA-DTT/PRT) Treatments May Benefit Specific ALDs

Social understanding–related ALDs			
Limited response to social rewards	Limited sharing of attention/ interests with others	Limited interest in peer relationships	Limited learning via imitation/ modeling
YES (via paired association)	No (attention directed to teaching materials)	No (object or teacher models)	**YES (via teaching incrementally, one step at a time)**
Communication-related ALDs			
Limited understanding of verbal/ nonverbal communication	Poor auditory processing speed/ discriminating words	Preference for visual over auditory recognition/ memory	Restricted perspective-taking/theory of mind
Partial (rotely learned and used only where directly taught)	Partial (telegraphic speech)	**YES (use of visuals and procedures)**	No (reliance on direct learning of expected response)
ALDs affecting play activities			
Lack of imagination	Eschews novelty/drawn to repetition	Sensory modulation difficulties	
Partial (rotely learned and used only where directly taught)	**YES (adult direction)**	**YES (step-by-step desensitization)**	

to offer, and where might they fit in with a multipronged approach to treatment? As you do research on treatment programs, you might get the feeling that proponents of ABA/DTT disrespect Floortime or RDI and vice versa. Understanding the differences will help you make your own judgment.

The strength of child-centric one-to-one treatment comes from focus on following the child's interests. The focus on child choice reduces battles for instructional control that can be so challenging in the early stages of adult-led one-to-one teaching, when the child does not yet understand (and accept) that he must "do something" to "get something." By following the child's lead, these interventions have the potential to desensitize the very slow-to-warm, anxious, or avoidant child to the overarousing aspects of social interactions. There are a number of child-centric approaches to treating autism, and we'll cover three common ones, exemplifying the potential advantages and drawbacks of child-centric treatment.

Hanen/Floortime/DIR and RDI

The Hanen Centre's "More Than Words" method, Stanley Greenspan and Serena Wieder's Floortime, and Steven Gutstein's RDI are three related approaches often used to treat toddlers and preschoolers with autism. *Hanen*, the term used most often to refer to work out of the Hanen Centre in Toronto, might best be described as a fusion of principles used by speech and language pathologists, behaviorists, and child psychiatrists—in that order. It is child-centric—it follows children's interests with principles like ROCK (R: Repeat what you say and do; O: Offer opportunities for the child to take a turn; C: Cue the child's turn; and K: Keep it fun). It is developmentally based, encouraging emerging language with the four S's: Say Less, Stress, Slow, and Show. It is less structured than PRT, more structured and didactic than Floortime. Hanen has not been marketed as aggressively as, say, RDI—which we'll get to in a minute—but because it promises less of a miracle, or it doesn't cost as much, doesn't mean it isn't a relevant method of child-centric intervention.

　　Floortime is the name most often used to refer to the therapeutic approach innovated by Greenspan and Wieder and more descriptively called the Developmental, Individual-differences, Relationship-based approach (or DIR). Greenspan is a child psychiatrist whose work on autism grew out of earlier work on temperamentally sensitive children and the fit between mother and child. That's why Floortime/DIR has such a big emphasis on sensory dysregulation—children with high reactivity to all sorts of changes can be particularly difficult for their parents to read and respond to. The idea behind Floortime is to build increasingly larger (more reciprocal, more sustained) "circles" of interaction between the child and the therapeutic adult. Treatment begins with simple two-way communication around something that is self-gratifying for the child, like playing with a simple toy, taking turns, and then adding twists to the turns so that the play requires just a little more attention and problem solving with each turn. For example, running a train along a track might be a starting point if this is what a particular child loves doing. The adult might watch for a while and then start saying "Go!" each time the train passes the station house. After a while, the adult might place her hand on the track, right before the station, and say "Stop!" and wait for the child to respond with "Go!" before letting the train continue. As the child's language and play capacities develop, increasingly symbolic interactions are introduced.

One underpinning for Floortime is the careful building of "circles" that help children with autism, who are often under- or overreactive to touch or certain noises, learn to anticipate triggers to sensory input, self-regulate, and eventually "exfoliate" these sensitivities. Shedding these sensitivities reveals a child with a capacity for more typical social reciprocity.

Floortime itself has not been subject to studies that compare its effectiveness to other approaches. (In fact there is almost no research that directly compares any of these methods to one another.) It is based on theory about how to help children with problems in self-regulation. Much of the evidence for Floortime's effectiveness comes from a case review study that its developers made on children who mostly had something they called "multisystem developmental disorder," or MSDD, which I mentioned in Chapter 3. Not that many doctors use MSDD as a diagnosis, but the kids who do receive it usually have the same hyper- and hyposensitivities that some children with an autism spectrum disorder also have (while not also qualifying for a diagnosis of an autism spectrum disorder). Because I view these sensitivities as a kind of ALD—meaning they interfere in specific ways with how a child may learn—Floortime may be a particularly good fit as part of an overall program for the autistic child who is not having much difficulty with language and is having relatively minor difficulties socially, especially with intensity of social overtures.

"Options" Therapy: Of Historical Interest

To the left of Floortime, we have Options—another child-led therapeutic approach for autism spectrum disorders. I am sometimes asked if Floortime is the same thing as Options. Options is a similar-looking intervention developed in the 1960s by parents of a then (reportedly) high-functioning child with autism. (I say reportedly because we did not have a concept of "high-functioning autism" in the sixties.) Although Options and Floortime have superficial commonalities, Floor-time is basically a specialized set of methods for what child psychia-trists would basically call "play therapy." Options, in contrast, is based on a more inspirational Rousseauian autistic-child-as-noble-savage idea: Parents mirror their child's actions—even things like hand flapping—in an effort to show the child that the parents' world is a safe place that the child can enter, guided by the parent. "Optioned" parents I've met have been "reeducated" in a way that undercuts their de facto unique expertise and qualifications to be part of their child's treatment team—and instead encourages them to overrely on the ex-pertise of the Options team. More important, of course, is that it doesn't seem to particularly "work" for autism, as "creating a safe place" is not where it's at for most children affected by symptoms of autism spectrum disorders.

Where Does RDI Come In?

About five years after Floortime first made a splash, RDI (Relationship Development Intervention) became a DIR-like "packaged" program that combined principles that Greenspan had gotten us thinking about. Steven Gutstein, RDI's innovator, pulled in the off-the-shelf merchan-dising that goes along with the DTT how-to manuals, combined it with about 10% Options inspirational messaging, added it to 80% Floortime, threw in 10% Hanen for good measure, and a "new" autism treatment was off and running. Often, RDI is marketed directly to par-ents through group seminars held in Texas, where Gutstein is based. It is certainly easier for parents to learn principles of RDI than of Floortime, though both really have the same underpinnings of follow-ing the child's lead into play as a way of sustaining engagement and intrinsically motivating the child. While this part is fine, as with Floortime, this can be more problematic for the younger or more se-verely affected child who "doesn't know what he doesn't know."

Where Parents Fit In

These child-centric approaches can be of great value to your child. They naturalize learning in a way that is just not part of DTT—no mat-ter what anyone tells you. There is no drill for spontaneity. Whatever approach you use as your main treatment, there is likely to be a point where you will also benefit from influences of more child-centric ap-proaches, even if you don't buy into one name brand or another. If you feel you must hook up with an RDI coach, then use him or her as a parent trainer. (For goodness' sake, don't spend thousands of dollars going to Texas for the weekend.) Have two to five sessions—preferably at home and not a therapist's office—helping you expand the natural teaching opportunities that occur in your home. Have the trainer coach you and perhaps also someone that you, or the therapist, feel can be good at applying these principles with your child in a natural manner. RDI (or any child-centric therapy) that just goes on in a therapist's office behind closed doors will not be nearly as powerful a treatment for your child as when you have a means to integrate it into your child's regular schedule. Child-centered therapy approaches are, like the adult-led approaches discussed first in this chapter, a matter of making your child's day-to-day living experiences part of his education and habilitation.

How Well Are ALDs Likely to Be Addressed?

So, is there room for child-led therapies in addressing how your child learns now? As in the table on page 158, you can see that these approaches don't do everything for everyone. You will need to decide whether a component of this sort of intervention would fit for your child now, as part of her treatment plan. Earlier, I suggested that DTTs can be a great initial approach to establishing instructional control. Similarly, these child-centric approaches might fit later, when the child has some established receptive language, emerging representational play, and so on. *The underlying message here is that as your child's profile of ALDs changes, so should the mix of treatments you use.*

Special Education Group-Based Approaches to Treating Autism

Okay, I've already said life is not one to one. This is one way of saying there is definitely a place for group-based special education classes for children with autism spectrum disorders. Being in a group helps children with more serious challenges learn the value of taking their cue from predictable routines and from others and function in a way that allows them to becoming increasingly independent. If you are a four-year-old girl with autism and are just starting to realize how fabulous it is to do something new by copying someone else, being in a group will have some advantages.

How One-to-One Child-Centered (Floortime/RDI/Hanen) Treatments May Benefit Specific ALDs

Social understanding–related ALDs			
Limited response to social rewards	Limited sharing of attention/ interests with others	Limited interest in peer relationships	Limited learning via imitation/ modeling
YES (via child choice of content)	YES (major focus)	No (adult as model for affiliation)	No (adult as model for affiliation)
Communication-related ALDs			
Limited understanding of verbal/ nonverbal communication	Poor auditory processing speed/ discriminating words	Preference for visual over auditory recognition/ memory	Restricted perspective-taking/theory of mind
YES (in context of social regulation)	No (often assumes receptive > expressive), except Hanen	YES (pairs words with activity)	YES (anticipation/ prediction of others' actions)
ALDs affecting play activities			
Lack of imagination	Eschews novelty/drawn to repetition	Sensory modulation difficulties	
YES (innovation as main focus	YES (innovation as main focus)	YES (gradual building of reciprocity	

When would it be wise to choose a special education group or classroom? Why *not* full inclusion? What about full inclusion with an aide? I'll discuss full inclusion, with and without an aide, starting on page 166, but first let me address why many parents think they don't want their child in special education. I have heard the "I don't want my child in a special ed class because then he'll learn to act like them" mantra many times. Where did this refrain come from? Are there data to support it? Actually, no. A child who doesn't yet imitate others is unlikely to imitate a bad behavior—at least not one that doesn't result in any positive consequences. (Autistic children, being instrumental learners, *will* learn successful bad behaviors that result in desired consequences. So if screaming gets you a back rub, and you like back rubs, you might try screaming too.) All things being equal, if a bad behavior is ignored or results in an undesired outcome, a child with autism will not learn it. Children don't learn their symptoms from each other. If your child doesn't imitate, she's not going to suddenly wake up one day in a TEACCH class, see someone flapping his hands, and think "Cool, I want to do that!" This stuff is hard-wired. What we're doing in treatment is *uncrossing* the wires.

I believe the desire not to place a child in special education is more emotional than rational—and understandably flows from an earnest desire to see your child as more typical and less atypical. But, if she could learn to be "normal" from just being around other kids, you wouldn't have been asked to remove her from two day care centers and a preschool before you went down the road to diagnosis.

One-to-One, Then Special Ed?

It often makes sense to think of a one-to-one program (adult-led or child-centric) as the first step that some children may need before they can move on to being part of a group. One-to one programs offer the opportunity to develop an awareness of another and accrue the potential benefits of taking turns in either teaching or play. However, for some children with a strong desire to follow routines, it might be easier to establish a motive to do certain things at certain times, in certain ways, or in a certain order in a classroom first, bypassing that bit about dealing one to one with someone else—which for some children with autism is a very big barrier.

The good news here is that increasingly schools offer hybrid programs that can flexibly offer one-to-one teaching (adult-led or child-centered) plus group-based teaching that plays to the desire for routine. What do these classes look like? First there is the classroom that is all one-to-one teaching or where a substantial part of the curriculum is administered one to one. Is "in-school" one-to-one as good for your child as at-home one-to-one? There's no evidence either way. But I like a little at-home one-to-one, at least at first, as it can be an important support for parent training.

One good reason to opt for a special day class over a general education class is when your child is not functioning at chronological age level with respect to receptive language. This means that a five-year-old who can listen only as well as a three-year-old is going to miss much of what's being said in general education kindergarten—which is already a setting where the teacher does more by "telling" than by "showing." If you're not up to the level of your peers, you're going to miss a lot, in terms of what other kids are saying and what they mean by what they are saying—not to mention in terms of your play interests, which are also likely to be quite "babyish" by five-year-old standards.

I am always amazed at how many parents buy into this idealized image of how other kindergarteners would like nothing more than to be a buddy to a child who doesn't really talk, doesn't know how to play their games, and might sometimes be aggressive. Of course, every class has one or two kids—the bossy five-year-old sister of twin two-year-olds, the cousin of a kid with Down syndrome—who really do want to be helpers and are good at it. This is great, but I can tell you that it's hard to see how many kids ignore yours, move away from him if and when they can, and do not act particularly altruistic.

More important, the whole idea of a peer who is an age-appropriate model needs to embrace a model at the developmental stage your child can "read." If he talks and plays like a three-year-old, this may be a preschool, or it may be a special day class where other five-year-olds are at the three-year developmental level.

TEACCH

The best-known, most well-established model for special day classes for children with autism is TEACCH. TEACCH stands for Treatment and Education of Autistic and related Communication-handicapped Children and was developed by Eric Schopler (also the founder of the *Journal of Autism and Developmental Disorders*) at the University of North Carolina. TEACCH is a comprehensive approach to families and children living with autism—much more comprehensive than just an educational method. It has programs that emphasize early identification, parent training, social and leisure skills development, and vocational training. TEACCH focuses on improving adaptive and independent living skills by modifying the environment to accommodate the characteristics of those with autism disorders.

TEACCH is built around the idea of making lemonade out of what you might have thought were lemons. Things we could see as weaknesses become strengths in navigating the world of a Project TEACCH program. If you love a routine, you've got it: A TEACCH class has a daily schedule with a predictable routine, an individual picture schedule ordering the major tasks of the whole day, visual prompts for ordering and completing work at the same individual workstation you use each day—lots and lots of routine. For the child who is preverbal or nonverbal, what's going to happen next becomes quickly predictable. For the child who is more visual than auditory, "seeing" what's happening makes so much more sense than just hearing about it. Other pupils encroaching on your space make you want to flap, hop, and vocalize like a tsunami early-warning system? No problem—in a TEACCH class you have your own little carrel, as isolated as you need it to be.

Quality Assurance

What is there not to like? Some would say it's *too* easy. There's not enough impetus to talk rather than to just cooperatively follow routines and follow pictured activities. A routine organized in fifteen-minute blocks can be carried off by an organized teacher. To me, a good TEACCH class is a good fit for many children with autism who are not yet (or, honestly, may never be) ready to be meaningfully and developmentally included with typically developing peers. But what makes a TEACCH class good? You may hear of many classes that are supposedly "TEACCH," but unless you live in and around North Carolina, they may be—or may not be. TEACCH does two-week summer institutes for already-credentialed teachers to certify them in TEACCH. This is a good training period. Many teachers are able to implement and transmit the TEACCH pedagogy after that. If a teacher has taken a two-day TEACCH training offered by her county office of education, she should have gotten the idea, but really will need to see a TEACCH class in action, read more, or get supervision to get things up and running. Of course, if she's the first one to implement this model in her area—that could be logistically difficult.

What's really good about TEACCH classes? They depend on lots of visuals. This is part of making lemonade with lemons: If a child is visual, you teach with pictures of exactly how he sees things—and explain things visually. (Of course, you use words too—so the words and pictures become meanings for the same thing.) However, some TEACCH classes increasingly rely on Mayer-Johnson icons—ready-made stick figures and line drawings that come on a CD-ROM. They are really convenient to use. However, no autistic child (no one, in fact) thinks in Mayer-Johnson icons, so a class that relies more heavily on photo icons, especially for its youngest and completely nonverbal pupils, is doing a better job playing to a child's autism-specific learning disabilities (ALDs).

Another thing that can be a nice innovation for a TEACCH class or any special day class is to borrow from general education preschool programs where children learn to put things away where they came from. At TEACCH class workstations, children do tasks in a row to earn a play break, dumping completed tasks into a "finished" basket or box below the workstation. This get-your-work-done-and-get-a-break concept quickly becomes motivating. However, when children have to replace task materials in meaningful locations around the classroom, they learn further skills that will be like what they will need to do in general education classes and as part of any daily living routine.

Some parents worry that TEACCH is not as "rapid-fire" as DTT, so their child will be learning less. On the contrary, there is research suggesting that instructional strategies where the child initiates the problem solving under his own steam, with less direct prompting, may be a key ingredient in developing a more independent learner. However, TEACCH workstations need at least two-to-one supervision, and children should never be allowed to just sit passive, unengaged with the task at hand. The adult should be stepping in to ensure that learning is a continuous process.

Is There a TEACCH Home Edition?

Can a TEACCH program be done at home? Certainly! If your child is very routine oriented, consider it part of her autistic learning style. It's your chance to make lemonade from the lemons of her otherwise irritating rigidity. Make it work for you—and for your child: Many parents successfully import picture schedules, visual schedules for particular activities, and even workstations to their homes. Some are used as an afterschool enrichment program, whereas some TEACCH features lend themselves to hybridization into everyday routines of any family—like getting dressed and then eating breakfast or setting the table in the evening.

I am also more often seeing and hearing about how TEACCH is being imported into the home by ABA providers who deliver a combination of discrete trial and PRT services. Some seem to feel the need to insist this isn't TEACCH but a part of ABA—but if it's going to potentially help your child, just stand clear of the ideological wars and let your provider roll it out.

The Special Day Class
That's Not Just for Children with Autism

Everything that is true of a good TEACCH special day class should be true of any good special day class. A special day class should be a place that can be tailored to your child's specific learning needs—which might be some DTT, some TEACCH, some child-centered play at break times. Some of the best special day classes I've seen combine these techniques, using discrete trial drills to introduce new material, TEACCH workstations to expand on concepts that have been introduced initially with discrete trials, and an adult in the "go play" break area who can expand on the child's play and language linked to his free choices. This means that such settings can often accommodate children with needs for different amounts of different kinds of treatment approaches.

However, in a more general special day class, it's important that children have somewhat comparable needs. This means that a class of six children, of whom two are low-functioning autistic children, two very high, and two in between, is probably not the best place for anyone. A teacher, no matter how good, is going to have a really hard time running three side-by-side classrooms—with different content, different pacing, different visual versus auditory strategies for getting information across. As a parent, you should seek out a class that can not only accommodate your child's autistic learning disabilities but also give him a place where he is more or less "in the middle." This means that most things that a child can learn from in the classroom are neither above nor below him.

Experiencing Independence

For some children, special day classes can be the first real step to becoming more independent learners. Special day classes can be small enough, developmentally accessible enough, and supported by sufficient staff to be ideal places to move away from full-time one-to-one supports—if that is the only learning experience the child has had up to that point. I've talked with some parents of children with autism who underestimate the importance of supporting their child to become more independent learners. If a particular child is ever going to succeed educationally in the mainstream, she'll need to take small steps getting there. The next small step after full-time one-to-one home-based programming is the small contained supported special day class with two-to-one or three-to-one small groups, some one-to-one teaching, and a limited amount of whole-group activity with a group of developmentally comparable peers.

Where Parents Fit In

So far, it's been pretty clear where you as a parent can help in one-to-one programs for your child. You basically slip right in there and start in where the paid staff leave off. You make the things the child is learning in her formal treatment hours "news to use" in the rest of her life. This adding of functional value provides a natural reinforcement that by definition is not there when you are just practicing (DTT) or playing (like Floortime).

There are two ways for parents to "wrap around" their child's special day class. The first is to be part of the class. The second is to do homework. Both of these strategies are extremely similar to what you would do for a child in any non-special-education class—only you need to be doing it from the preschool years on.

Parents in the Classroom

In some schools, school administrators now have a healthy dose of concern when parents want to visit the class: This is because there are parents who have been known to sit at the back of the class, taking notes on this or that, and then days later hit the district with a notice of hearing for due process. Not nice. Yes, I've heard the horror stories. Yes, I've lived through some horror stories. Yes, I have testified about the horrors. I have also testified about how such alleged horrors might not be so horrible if you only knew why a teacher was or wasn't doing what she is doing. Going into a classroom mainly to dig dirt is more than a little disingenuous as a way to best help your child. I take the approach that you're not in much of a position to criticize if you haven't been there *and* done that—in other words, put your money where your mouth is.

I know you can read websites that encourage you to drop in to your child's special education class unannounced. Have you ever heard of a parent of a general education child who does that? No—

99.9% of parents have too much dignity and too much respect for the school as the institution responsible for educating children and for the teacher to whom their child is entrusted. This should be the starting point in special education classes too.

What should you do then? How about volunteer? We have lots of parents who volunteer in day care and preschool co-ops, as well as elementary classes. This gives you an opportunity to learn more about your child via his similarities with and differences from classmates and what does or doesn't work for them. It allows you to try out some of the techniques you see, while being coached by professionally trained staff. These are all the same reasons you might volunteer in a general education class. Importantly, you get the feel of how hard or easy it is to make the magic of a "teaching moment" and a "learning moment" so you can get an additional perspective on what's going on.

Homework

As far as homework and children on the autistic spectrum go, it would be hard for me to say whether the children or the parents dislike it more. Often homework that consists of worksheets that extend the school day are bilaterally hated. Maybe, just maybe, that's not what homework should be. Just as we discussed with respect to "wraparound" work for parents with children in one-to-one programs, children in group programs need the same thing. Talk to the teacher about a school-to-home daily log book that notes new vocabulary, activities, and materials as well as suggestions about how related activities at home might make these things more meaningful as they continue to be taught in school. These can be simple things: If a child is learning barnyard animal names, maybe a trip to a petting zoo. If a child is learning to count, maybe some water play dumping cups with numbers and related quantities. An older or more advanced child studying weather might watch the Weather Channel for specific information.

How Well Are ALDs Likely to be Addressed?

TEACCH classes play to many aspects of the autistic learning style and provide accommodation for a range of ALDs: Special day classes, unlike other specific program models, are more of a carte blanche to write in whatever is needed. On page 166, as for the other treatment models we've discussed, is some help in organizing your thoughts on how well features of a TEACCH class or any special day class with some of

How Special Education (TEACCH/ Other Special Day Classes) May Benefit Specific ALDs

Social understanding–related ALDs			
Limited response to social rewards	**Limited sharing of attention/ interests with others**	**Limited interest in peer relationships**	**Limited learning via imitation/ modeling**
No (completed order as reward)	No (attention directed to routine or materials)	No (inclusion with comparable peers)	No (routine as model)
Communication-related ALDs			
Limited understanding of verbal/ nonverbal communication	**Poor auditory processing speed/ discriminating words**	**Preference for visual over auditory recognition/ memory**	**Restricted perspective-taking/theory of mind**
Partial (routine as replacement)	No (emphasis on visual)	**YES (visually sequenced environment)**	No (work is individual)
ALDs affecting play activities			
Lack of imagination	**Eschews novelty/drawn to repetition**	**Sensory modulation difficulties**	
No (more emphasis on classification)	**YES (delimited tasks)**	**YES (controlled physical environment)**	

these features may mesh with your child's specific autistic learning profile.

Approaches to Treating Autism in General Education Settings

It goes without saying that all parents wish their child "belonged" in general education and not special education. Wishing does not make it so—though the law does. In this section, we'll do some wrestling with the countervailing forces of inclusion as a civil right versus inclusion as a choice based on the child's specific ALDs and ALSs and aimed at what's best developmentally and educationally for the child.

The Terms *Mainstreaming* and *Inclusion*

There are many kinds of inclusion. In the past, the term *mainstreaming* was used to describe children who had been in special education and were being assisted to enter the "mainstream"—namely, regular education classes. The term *inclusion* is often now used preferentially or interchangeably with *mainstreaming*. Inclusion can be full (for the whole school day) or partial—meaning the child is assigned a special day class but also a general education class, where he typically spends more and more of his time as certain benchmarks are reached. There are also hybrid programs, especially in preschool programs, that are referred to as *integrated*, meaning some of the pupils have an IEP and some don't—because they are developing typically. (I do not use the hideous term *neurotypical*—it's like implying that having a problem is just as okay as not having a problem.)

Inclusion

There are many potential advantages to consider when deciding whether some (or full) inclusion is part of the treatment formula your child needs. One appealing thing is that the child is educated in his immediate community, often his neighborhood. Classmates can be neighbors. Parents may be families similar to your own. Making play dates can be relatively easy. For the child who has some home- and some school-based services, a local school usually means less of a commute between the two parts of the treatment. The next table shows how and when an inclusive placement may be beneficial in addressing your child's ALDs.

Full Inclusion

What would you say would be the number-one advantage of putting your child in full inclusion? Most parents would say "She'll be with age-appropriate role models." True. But will she be ready to learn from them? Think of it this way: If you have a very smart five-year-old who multiplies and divides, will she learn calculus without learning alge-

How General Education (Full or Partial Inclusion) May Benefit Specific ALDs

Social understanding–related ALDs			
Limited response to social rewards	Limited sharing of attention/ interests with others	Limited interest in peer relationships	Limited learning via imitation/ modeling
No (response assumed)	YES (once imitation present)	YES (if peers are interesting models)	YES (if salient peer models)
Communication-related ALDs			
Limited understanding of verbal/ nonverbal communication	Poor auditory processing speed/ discriminating words	Preference for visual over auditory recognition/ memory	Restricted perspective-taking/theory of mind
No (assumed mastered)	No (assumed mastered)	No (assumed mastered)	YES (via group participation)
ALDs affecting play activities			
Lack of imagination	Eschews novelty/drawn to repetition	Sensory modulation difficulties	
Partial (if child imitates and at developmental level)	Partial (varied curriculum if child can follow it)	No (environment designed for those without difficulty)	

bra if she's put with kids who are ready to learn it? Of course not. Kids cannot skip stages. Language is not a behavior. Play is not a behavior. Because these are developmentally organized skills, children proceed through an organized set of stages to get from point A to point Z.

Partial Inclusion

For many children, a good way to start education in the mainstream is a little bit at a time. If your child has been in an ABA program, you have probably gotten the idea that things are learned in small increments. If a child cannot succeed at a task put before him, he is prompted to complete one part of the task (say a puzzle), then two, then three, till the whole is completed. If you were a very good teacher who was teaching this child to do the puzzle, you might start by helping him put in the circle piece of the puzzle if you knew he already recognized "circle" and could do it on other puzzles, working up to the weirdest, most unfamiliar shapes.

Think of inclusion and starting with partial inclusion the same way. Start a little bit at a time, consolidating success and starting at the place the child is most likely to succeed. If you have a six-year-old with autism who reads expressively at the third grade level but is still much further behind on using his language to talk to other children, a good idea would be to start him in a first-grade reading group. Even if he doesn't yet chatter much with the other kids, if they think he's the best reader in their reading group, they'll have a reason to admire and like him. On the other hand, if his first inclusion experience is recess, and he never answers other kids who verbally or gesturally try to invite him to play, he'll be relatively less appealing. Research on the development of peer relations among typically developing children shows that peers perceived as more aggressive or noncompliant or hyperactive than others tend not to be as well liked as peers who are not.

Quality Assurances

If you are wondering whether your child is ready for some mainstreaming, and whether it will afford her an opportunity to learn in new ways, here are some considerations to help you decide whether it's time yet.

The Egocentric World of the Three-Year-Old

First, how old is your child chronologically? If she is under five and you are thinking of including her with agemates, particularly three- or four-year-olds, a major consideration is that even typically developing children under four or five have relatively undeveloped capacities for perspective-taking themselves. This means, if another three-year-old invites your child to play and your child does not respond immediately, it will be taken as a no. Three-year-olds "revise." A three-year-old doesn't circle back, give it another go, try to make sure your child is listening and understanding; he'll just look for someone else on the playground who can provide more immediate gratification. Now, a five-year-old will. He will flip into "big brother" mode and cajole and coax, especially if encouraged by an adult—or if there is no other game in town. This tells us that large free-play groups of preschool agemates are not likely the best first inclusion experience.

Dress for Success

This brings us to a second parameter: setting up opportunities for your child to be successful. Another rule as you start to think about including your child in a mainstream class is that if you start him at something relatively structured, and something he's relatively on par at, he will need less one-to-one prompting. Certainly from kindergarten on, classmates are completely tuned in to who a one-to-one extra adult in a class is shadowing. This does not help make your child pass as a "regular guy." Some kids are attracted to the aide and the extra adult attention that can accrue—which is great for your child—but this is a qualitatively different kind of peer experience than other kids in the class have when they choose to learn incidentally from one another.

Making Inclusion "Real"

If your child is not within developmental "arm's reach" of peers with respect to any of the aspects of the classroom day, inclusion may not offer incremental benefit at this point. A capacity for imitation and a desire to be with and do things with peers, as well as developmental models your child can access, are all critical prerequisites to successful inclusion.

It is, however, possible to include just about any child. I have even seen a child in a general education class seated in a confined area in the back and given DTT for two hours each day—and then sent home. Are molecules promoting typical development supposed to be floating back there and helping somehow? What you want to avoid is the classroom-within-a-classroom phenomenon, where your child has a completely different set of requirements for fulfilling the tasks of the school day—it's a further barrier to peers providing meaningful models.

Resource Specialist Programs

Do you think your child may be ready for inclusion some of the time, but not all of the time? If you have a child who presents no real disruptive behaviors that interfere with his ability to learn, and he also can function "within arm's reach" developmentally for some subjects in the inclusion classroom—like reading and math—this may be your very best alternative. But what about when he "fries"—when he can take only two hours of a three-and-a-half-hour school day?

Some schools might suggest a special day class "homeroom" where he starts and perhaps finishes his school day. For some pupils, this may be fine if they can slide on into the routine—because they've been with this teacher in previous years or know the other kids or know the classroom and its routines. If the child is just starting school for the first time, a resource room may be an important educational resource to consider instead of a special day class.

What's a Resource Room?

Resource rooms—or simply "resource" in many schools—are a kind of floating special education classroom, usually staffed by an experienced special education teacher who has taught many different things and many different kinds of children. A resource room looks like an after-school tutoring center—computers, curriculum materials, and bulletin boards on many different subjects at many different levels. General education pupils are usually assigned "resource" to get extra help on math or reading. Higher-functioning pupils with autism often have "resource" for group-based social skills, conversation, or language pragmatics groups in addition to academic subjects. "Resource" can focus on specific subjects. Another good use of a resource room is for one-to-one "preteaching" of an activity that will come up soon in your child's general education class, so the newness and faster pacing alone do not "throw" him. Some resource time is in small groups of two or three pupils, and this can be really helpful for the child who comes to general education after nothing but full-time one-to-one home schooling.

Matching ALDs to Treatment Approaches

The table on pages 172 and 173 simply turns the previous four inside out: Each of the areas of autistic learning disability we originally talked about in Chapter 6 are cross-tabulated side by side with each of the four kinds of comprehensive approaches to treating autism that we've covered in this chapter. The point is that no one treatment really seems to tackle every area where a child with autism may be having difficulty

Area of ALD	One-to-one adult-led (ABA-DTT/PRT)	One-to-one child-centric (Floortime/Hanen/RDI)	Special education (TEACCH/other special day class)	General education (full or partial inclusion)
Social understanding–related ALDs	**Primary likely benefits**			
Limited response to social rewards	**YES** (via paired association)	No (completed order as reward)	**YES** (via child choice of content)	No (response assumed)
Limited sharing of attention/interests with others	No (attention directed to teaching)	No (attention directed to routine or materials)	**YES** (major focus)	**YES** (once imitation present)
Limited interest in peer relationships	No (object or teacher models)	No (inclusion with comparable peers)	No (adult as model for affiliation)	**YES** (if peers are interesting models)
Limited learning via imitation/modeling	**YES** (via teaching incrementally, one step at a time)	No (routine as model)	No (adult as model for affiliation	**YES** (if salient peer models)
Communication-related ALDs	**Primary likely benefits**			
Limited understanding of verbal/nonverbal communication	Partial (rotely taught/non-generative)	Partial (routine as replacement)	**YES** (in context of social regulation)	No (assumed mastered)
Poor auditory processing speed/discriminating words	Partial (telegraphic speech)	No (emphasis on visual)	No (often assumes receptive > expressive)	No (assumed mastered)

Area of ALD	One-to-one adult-led (ABA-DTT/PRT)	One-to-one child-centric (Floortime /Hanen/ RDI)	Special education (TEACCH /other special day class)	General education (full or partial inclusion)
Communication-related ALDs	Primary likely benefits			
Preference for visual over auditory recognition/ memory	YES (use of visuals and procedures)	YES (visually sequenced environment)	YES (pairs words with activity)	No (assumed mastered)
Restricted perspective-taking/theory of mind	No (reliance on direct learning)	No (work is individual)	YES (anticipation/ prediction of others' actions)	YES (via group participation)
ALDs affecting play activities	Primary likely benefits			
Lack of imagination	Partial (rotely taught/non-generative)	No (more emphasis on classification)	YES (innovation as main focus)	Partial (if child imitates and at developmental level)
Eschews novelty/ drawn to repetition	YES (adult direction)	YES (delimited tasks)	YES (innovation as main focus)	Partial (varied curriculum if child can follow it)
Sensory modulation difficulties	YES (desensitization)	YES (controlled physical environment)	YES (gradual building of reciprocity)	No (environment designed for those without difficulty)

learning. Look at this table and think about the first column. Where are your child's learning difficulties the greatest?

If you filled out the informal rating scale for these that was suggested in Chapter 6, put those numbers into the corresponding boxes in the first column of this table. Now look at which treatment does best on the things you rated as your child's biggest barriers to learning. What does the preponderance of the evidence tell you about which treatment should be the one you emphasize most strongly? Are there areas where you definitely need coverage that this "first choice" doesn't cover or doesn't cover well? What does cover them? Add some of that too. This type of analysis should give you some perspective on how much you need of what.

Remember that the "mix" you select should never be seen as fixed in stone. Once you start, you can shift based on how your child does. This is why educators call an IEP an *individualized* education program. This is why we set benchmarks (called *objectives* on an IEP) that can be points for revisiting what actually has been learned and then what to teach next. This will be discussed more in Part IV of this book, when we get into the mechanics of working with schools and public agencies that pay for treatment. Suffice it to say for now that public schools do pay for all the kinds of programs we have discussed in this chapter. Strategically, it's a matter of working with what's available in terms of programs, working with evaluators who can guide you with respect to your child's strengths (ALSs) and weaknesses (ALDs), and putting them together to make your child's IEP.

How Much Is Enough?

Yes, we've already addressed this question in this book. But when I meet with parents of children with autism about treatment planning, there are days I wish I had a button for my blazer that said "It's not about the number of hours!" The question comes up throughout the diagnostic and treatment process, so I'm answering it again here.

What you should want is a program with *content* that is geared developmentally to what your child needs to learn next. This is true irrespective of which main treatment method you adopt. The treatment methods are just that—*methods.* The *content* is what is most crucial. By analogy, it's not whether you drive a car with a stick shift or an automatic transmission—it's where you go that counts. If the content of what is being taught is over your child's head (because he's not yet ready for the prerequisites), it will not matter how many hours a day of program he has. In college, we don't let students take Quantum Physics before taking Physics I. A child who does not spontaneously speak in single words should not be prompted to emit three-word sentences. It will make no more sense to him than string theory does to me— because I've never even taken Physics I.

Making sure that the curriculum content is developmentally appropriate is absolutely crucial. This is what time in an IEP meeting should be spent on—as far as I'm concerned. Too often it's all about "which services" and "how many hours"—with less attention to what teachers and therapists will actually teach during those hours. Your job as "general contractor" is to make sure good-quality materials are used. In this case, this means that if your three-year-old tests with eighteen-month receptive language (which might be measured by something like good noun recognition for everyday objects), the next thing to teach is two-year-old language (like action words to attach to those nouns: "*Bye-bye*, Daddy," or "Juice *all gone*"), If you try to skip from "juice" to "I want juice, please," ignoring the innate building blocks of language, you'll be training a behavior, not promoting a vocabulary of concepts that can grow to be flexibly, spontaneously interchanged (like the child spontaneously coming up with "*my* juice," "Daddy car bye-bye").

Assuming that the curriculum is developmentally geared to what your child needs to learn next, you can then begin to think of criteria that determine intensity as measured by the numbers of hours in treatment. For very young children entering treatment for the first time, two important criteria are (1) resistance to treatment and (2) nap times. Some children are passive and tolerate demands and retrials pretty readily. Some children are quickly pleased to learn that they have discovered a way to get what appears to be unfettered access to favorite foods and cooperate readily with whatever you step them through. Then, though, are the my-way-or-the-highway guys. These are the little ones who heretofore have been accustomed to doing what they want, when they want, how they want, for as long or as much as they want. Initiation of any treatment is a big irritation for them. By pushing too hard, adding too many hours too quickly, you run the risk of getting such a child turned off to teachers and the whole process of learning rather than seeing teaching sessions as an opportunity for things to be broken down in such a way that they eventually make more sense. It can be difficult to tell before starting treatment how hard it will be for any particular child to tolerate. Fortunately, IFSPs (individualized family service plans—the Early Start counterpart of IEPs), IEPs, therapists, and agencies of all sorts, plus preschools and special day classes, are pretty much used to this. Starting slowly with two half-hour sessions for a particularly stubborn fellow might be fine. By the end of a week of daily work of that sort, two forty-five-minute sessions might well be possible. After a month, a couple of forty-five-minute sessions separated by a brief but restorative break could work. After another month, two hours in the morning, two in the afternoon could be tried. My general experience is that if you push too hard at the very beginning, you'll lose more time having to back off and then ramp up again more slowly. This type of timing is easier to manage with home programs than ones at school. At school, having individual staff support so a child can be removed from a group for more free play can be a way of taking breaks from the curriculum.

Getting started, however, is a very individual thing. Some children just eat up the chance to be part of a predictable, structured learning activity. Such children, even very young ones, may be fine with a couple of hours consecutively (with small breaks) from the beginning, even when twenty-two to twenty-four months old.

Very young children are another case. Knowing how to structure a program for children under eighteen months old is not simple. You don't just do what you'd do with a three-year-old. Would you put a sixteen-month-old in a preschool class with three-year-olds? As for all young toddlers, whose world is naturally very self-centered, more child-centric approaches make developmental sense. Physical stamina increases with age too. Perhaps one of the most awful home program videos I ever saw was of a sixteen-month-old who had been "diagnosed" at thirteen months old and was being given a DTT program— much as if she was two years older. In between trials she lay on her back in her crib, sucked her thumb, held her blanket, and tried to sleep with the TV on—presumably to offer her some "downtime" stimulation. It looked like torture to me, and she certainly looked like one unhappy little cookie.

Learning should be fun for your child—though he may not be happy for every moment. Look for those "Ah-ha!" moments when you see that enlightenment of coming to understand something new. Look for that intense gaze of concentration as active problem solving is going on. Those are the purest moments of learning. Gear your child's "hours" to get as many of those moments as you can.

Adding On the à la Carte Selections

Remember, no one approach does everything for anyone: Which comprehensive treatment, how much of it you need, and what is developmentally appropriate curriculum content take you much of the way there. In Chapter 8, you can look for additional strategies that specifically target areas of your child's ALDs that your comprehensive program may not or that supplement your main treatment approach's offerings—or that may simply be fun and enriching in a way that helps your child learn to love learning.

EIGHT

The Customized Course

ADDITIONAL STRATEGIES
THAT TARGET SPECIFIC NEEDS

In Chapter 7 you should have gotten a pretty good idea of which parts of which of the core, comprehensive treatments for autism will help your child. You may have a fairly clear picture of how much of each of these approaches your child should get at this time. Because you have a solid grasp of what your child's autism-specific learning deficits (ALDs) and learning styles are, you might even be prepared to advocate for shifts in the ratio of treatments as you observe your child's progress.

What you've been doing is plotting the best general course—the route between point A and point B—for your particular child. Or you've been choosing the most satisfying-looking fixed-price menu. Whatever metaphor you apply, you undoubtedly recognize that making the broad decisions—mapping a route "as the crow flies" or picking out a fixed-price meal—isn't going to get you everything you want for your son or daughter. You'll want to add some à la carte choices to your meal, or depart occasionally from the well-traveled road to get exactly the help your child needs.

The goal is to make a complete list of the things you'll want to ask for to address *all* your child's learning difficulties when it comes time to go to that IEP meeting for your child. We'll talk about how to be effective at that meeting in the next chapter. But first, in this chapter, I'll help you take what you know about how your child learns and match it with strategies that specifically target the biggest barriers to learning for children with autism:

- Motivation
- Behaviors incompatible with paying attention and learning
- Communication, including increasing spontaneous communicating
- Social skills

As I stressed in the last chapter, choosing the right "name brand" methods for your child's learning style will make a lot of difference, but ensuring that the content is developmentally "what comes next" will make *all* the difference in whether he can benefit as much as possible from the methods selected. What comes next means what typically developing children learn next. What's different for your child should be not "what comes next" in terms of content but the age at which the teaching happens, the amount of rehearsal that may be needed, the motivators you will need to use, and the ALDs that will need to be accommodated.

Does your child need lots of help controlling behaviors that stand in the way of learning in more formal settings? Does she need to be better motivated to make those small but steady steps in development? Are current motivational strategies not powerful enough to be consistently effective? Are there areas of communication and social skills that demand focus beyond what the core program provides? If you answered yes to one or more of these questions, read on to get ideas of some additional strategies you can discuss with your child's prospective or current treatment providers. Also, it's important to know that each of these areas is one where the best results are achieved when parents "wrap around" efforts at school or therapy so that demands and expectations for increasingly mature behavior are made on your child wherever he finds himself.

How to Boost Motivation

Motivation is key. It doesn't matter whether you're asking "How do I make my child more interested in learning?" or "How do I make my child more interested in the rest of his family?" or "How do I make my child more interested in communicating?" Motivation is the key. This is where we'll start.

In the last chapter, I said one of the strengths of ABA (applied behavior analysis) programs is that primary reinforcers (like a highly desired food) are paired with social praise. As a child does something you want him to do again—put a piece in a puzzle, say a word in response to a model, or get up off the floor—you help him through it, give him a bit of desired food, and tell him he's great and you're proud of him. Soon, as he understands what's expected, you can "fade" the food, and lo and behold, the verbal praise has just the same effect. (That's classical conditioning.) How do we tailor and nuance this very fundamental learning principle?

Developing a Reward Hierarchy

A reward hierarchy is simply a list you make (and share) with everyone who works with your child. It's a list of what your child cares about. Some love Buzz Lightyear, others SpongeBob SquarePants—no accounting for taste. Some kids will initially work only for preferred foods. For others, the most rewarding things are sensory, such as squishy things to hold or twirl, tickles, or bubbles blown in the face. Make a list of what it is for your child. Pay no attention to what "should" be rewarding. Teaching *your* child begins where *your* child is at. You as the parent are key here. You know your child and what matters to him. There is no rewarding him with M&Ms if he hates chocolate.

A reward hierarchy is not only a list of what your child likes but also should reflect the order of importance of these items. It should also reflect how these items can be titrated. An M&M is easy—one M&M for one good deed. (I prefer the baking M&Ms because they are smaller—and because I personally prefer dark to milk chocolate, and even a teacher or therapist needs a reward once in a while for working hard.) Videos, on the other hand, are a lousy reward, because if you try to turn one on and then off again fifteen seconds later, you'll cause more problems than the reward is worth. For young learners, having to wait for a reward is hard to understand and even harder to accept. The rewarding needs to keep pace with the effort being expended.

Teaching Persistence

Rewards should be meted out according to effort. When you're teaching something new, trying is as important as succeeding. Success on even an approximation of a new, not-yet-mastered task is valuable. It shows the child that problem solving is a valuable skill—just as having a problem solved is a valuable goal. The way you might think about it is that persisting is just as desirable as successful problem solving. When you see a teacher you think is a great teacher, it's probably because she is making learning fun. She is helping your child learn to enjoy problem solving.

Parents can be upset when they see their child perseveratively doing something simple (like lining up crayons end to end)—over and over. Think about it. One reason this is upsetting is that it's showing you your child has not learned that persisting at solving a new challenge can feel good. Learning to persist at a task is a critical skill. If the child is ever going to be a "self-starter" and attack new cognitive challenges on her own, the act of problem solving must become self-gratifying. As a child masters a task, though, a reward needs to be held out for the real effort. As a parent, you will need to work with anyone starting to work with your child to ensure that he or she can do this effectively and efficiently.

On the other hand, a teacher or therapist new to your child may be able to bring her experience to bear and demonstrate a couple of new tricks for getting your child to persist on task and follow through on problem solving. (All children are very good at training parents to do as much for them as possible while putting in as little effort of their own as possible. Children with autism can be real masters at this.)

Another important aspect of reinforcement is doing it quickly enough so that it is clearly associated with the desired behavior or "good try" you want to see more often. The best example of this that I can give is in the use of token economies—like "sticker" charts where the child must do the desired thing (like peeing in the potty) some number of times (with a sticker for each) before the "real" reward (like a new Thomas train) is earned. This may work in school, where your child gets a sticker for each of three completed worksheets and then earns a play break on the trampoline. At home, though, where there are likely many more fun things to do than sit on the potty, more immediate and salient reinforcement is likely to be needed to motivate potty use. (The method I like is letting the child see but not yet have a very desirable toy enclosed in a clear plastic jar while sitting on the potty, giving the child immediate—but brief—play time with the toy in the bathroom right after a successful potty trip.)

Discovering New Reinforcers

There's a lot more to theory about reinforcement than we can cover here.* What's important here is to understand your role in specifying what your child finds rewarding. These rewards will change over time. As you discover new rewards, sharing them with those who teach your child is invaluable. Try to expand the list of things that are rewarding so your child doesn't get tired of the things he likes. If Buzz Lightyear is great, maybe some of that magic can wear off on Woody; if it's SpongeBob SquarePants, maybe that stupid little starfish can come to be admired as well.

Why Should I Care?

Whenever you teach something to a child with autism, picture a little cartoon thought bubble over his head. If, during an instructional task, play activity, or request for participation, the thought bubble says, "Why should I care?" you need to stop and make the activity something worth caring about (see the cartoon on page 183). You *can* always use a primary reinforcer—something from your reinforcer hierarchy. The name of the game, however, is to work a bit harder and make the reward *intrinsically meaningful* to the task. If you're a child who loves tickles, it is going to be easier to learn to distinguish pictures of dogs from pictures of cats if a stuffed dog tickles you whenever you identify a dog picture. After a while, also having the child name the body part to be tickled before the reinforcer is administered makes dogs, tickles, and body parts all the more interesting. Stuffed dogs and real dogs might even be added to the reinforcer hierarchy.

---

*There's more in my book *Helping Children with Autism Learn* (see Resources at the end of this book).

How Families Help

If, at this point, you've been exposed to ABA/DTT programs, you may have seen how continually extrinsic reinforcers are used. By "extrinsic" reinforcers I mean reinforcers that have nothing inherently to do with the success the child has achieved—like a food snack or a tickle. This works, but what does it mean for how you should be encouraging your child's development (and leveraging the value of her therapies) during after-therapy hours? I would not suggest that you do more drills. Reading your child a story at night after working with flash cards with dogs during the day can do the "dog tickle" part. If your child has also "studied" body parts, you can be the one to get her to label a stuffed animal and then label where it tickles her. It doesn't have to be structured. Rather, it should be natural and spontaneous. It's just that it requires a lot more nuance, spontaneous creativity, and a pretty thorough knowledge of your child's emerging skills. The very best therapists do figure out how to fit strategies like this into their everyday teaching. But you have great daily opportunities to make drill vocabulary into "news you can use" after the therapists go home or after your child comes home from school.

If you want to motivate your child to learn, here, in summary, are the key questions to keep asking yourself:

- "Am I reinforcing him with something he likes?"
- "Am I doing it often enough for it to matter to her?"
- "Am I asking him to do something he can see a reason to care about?"
- "Am I using a reinforcer that has some meaning intrinsic to the thing being taught" (like a tickle to the tummy for identifying "tummy")?

How to Address Problem Behavior

The flip side of motivating positive behavior is deterring problem behavior. Problem behavior can really be classified in one of three ways:

- Behavior that interferes with learning
- Behavior that is disruptive to others
- Behavior that injures the child

Consistency Isn't the Hobgoblin of Small Minds

If you're to help your child with autism learn, a key role is managing the behaviors that interfere with his ability to learn. It's not a job just for teachers when the child is in school or therapists when the child is in therapy. Remember, the child with autism is, above all, an instrumental learner. He is looking for the easiest way to have what he wants. If he has to do it one way with others but can still get away with an easier way with parents, he will. For the child to become an adaptable learner, experiencing a consistent, highly predictable world where the rules are the same everywhere makes things more comprehensible in the long run.

Getting a Child Ready to Learn

Children who aren't paying attention are not going to be able to learn. A good deal of inattention can come from not understanding language, but your child may also distract himself intentionally when experiencing the discomfort of a sensory overreaction, such as by covering his ears to certain sounds. Or he may just space out when underresponsive to other sensory input. Maybe he focuses his attention on making repetitive movements when overexcited or, conversely, when bored—or he simply has a strong drive to do things repetitively, which narrows opportunities for exploration and the possibility of new input. Kids with autism also often visually scrutinize certain things closely while ignoring the "bigger picture." When these behaviors stand between the child and something you'd like him to learn, you have good reason to want to eliminate them. They can all be modified when a functional behavioral analysis (often referred to as an FBA) is conducted. You may have heard this term. It may sound offputtingly technical, but you can and should learn basically what this is all about so you can team with professionals who will need to know from you when your child is and is not most likely to be engaged.

The ABCs of FBAs

A functional behavior analysis uses principles of ABA to systematically examine an undesired behavior and figure out what causes it and how to stop it or redirect a response to be more functional for the child. Think of your child's most annoying behavior. Okay, now know that getting rid of it can be as simple as ABC.

A stands for "antecedents." What happens just *before* the annoying behavior starts? *B* stands for "behavior"—the thing you wish never to see again. *C* stands for "consequences"—whatever results after the behavior occurs. Here's an example: Rogue, the four-year-old offspring of a laid-back California surfer dude and dudette, was a first-class screamer. (Rogue is not his real name—but his real name means the same thing.) Rogue often emitted unbearably high-pitched shrieks. Shrieking in this case is "B"—the "behavior." What is "C"—the "consequence"? His parents dropped everything else to figure out what he wanted. So, the "antecedent" was Rogue's having a need; the "behavior" was Rogue shrieking; and the "consequence" was his parents' prompt attention to the need state. If I were Rogue, the little thought bubble over my head would say, "Why should I stop?" He had a system that worked for him.

How Families Help

When a child has a behavioral problem like Rogue's—clearly one that interferes with learning and is disruptive to others—an FBA will be needed. Shrieking was a quick, easy, and effective way to say "I want something." It was much harder for Rogue to say *what* he wanted—though he could. His parents were directed to respond to shrieking only by offering choices—including something Rogue might not like: "Juice?" "Snack?" "TV off?" If there was no affirmative answer, juice was offered; if there was still no answer, the TV was turned off. If the shrieking continued, Rogue got a short time-out in his room, then new choices were offered again. When any words rather than shrieks were used to make a request, the request was met. This type of situation is exactly where you have a critical role in partnering with the "behavior analyst" in changing your child's patterns. Parents are more often in a better position than the professional doing the FBA to suggest possible antecedents and predicted consequences to the behavior targeted for change. You're the ones who know what the child probably means by what he says and does—even if he's not "saying" or "doing" in a way we'd like to see.

As a parent, you need to work with the behavior analyst or behavioral specialist to identify behaviors you see as interfering with attending and learning, as hurting others or self, or as interfering with any aspect of functioning. You need to share with the professional your best understanding of what sets these behaviors rolling. When can you anticipate your child will "toast"? What stories can you tell that illustrate situations where undesirable behaviors happen? This type of dialogue with the behavior analyst can really help fine-tune your child's FBA.

The behaviorist's job is to watch the child, see the behavior that's targeted as problematic, collect his own data on what antecedents he sees (to confirm, add to, or modify your list), and come up with new consequences. If the consequence works in eliminating the behavior when the behaviorist tries it, the consequence will work when you try it too. That's the good news. The bad news is that when the behavior is "consequenced" by the behaviorist and *not* by you, you are pretty much guaranteed the behavior will be just as bad when you're around. So, for example, if Rogue's behaviorist implemented 100% insistence on "using your words" and his parents did not, we would expect shrieking around his parents to continue. Obviously, then, you as parents are critical "active ingredients" in your child's overall success.

Getting Everyone on the Same Page (Grandma Too)

To get any child to change a bad behavior that "works" for him is hard. To get a child with autism to change bad behavior is harder. Since children with autism often rely more on experiential and procedural cues, you're unlikely to "talk" them out of anything. This means when you work with a behaviorist to develop a "behavioral plan"—the way to change the antecedents or consequences—you need to be prepared to come on board as an implementer of the plan. If the antecedent of some shrieking might be thirst, you're going to need to be ready to help the behaviorist come up with some simple way of teaching your child to ask for a drink. Let's say the behaviorist devises a plan for you to show your shrieking child a picture of his sippy cup, hold it to your mouth while you say, "Cup?!" "Cup!?"—and then give your child his sippy cup if his behavior changes in a way that lets you know you've got things right. With a plan like this, you and the behaviorist might decide that over time the child must hand you the picture himself to get you to hold it up and say "Cup." Once you decide what to do, *everybody* in your child's life must be shown how to do this and stick to it. This includes you—100% of the time. It also includes Grandma, who feels satisfying hunger or thirst on any demand is her entitlement as a grandma. And *you* must tell Grandma that if she really wants to help her grandchild, *she* needs to follow the new rules too—also 100% of the time. You, the parent, as "enforcer" of teaching demands on your child, are the cement that holds any kind of treatment plan together. Only you as a parent can perform this function that is so critical to your child's treatment success. Only you are with him all the time—not the best behaviorist in the world.

Besides coming up with the FBA, the behaviorist should be your support in being as close to 100% consistent with this as possible. No one can be 100% all the time, but being only 75% or 80% consistent with new demands will intermittently make the behavior you are trying to reduce get worse, and you might end up with an even worse problem than the one you started with. In addition, most children will go through an "extinction burst" when expectations for a new behavior are first put in place. This means they will try to use the bad behavior more—just to make sure they really can't get it to work. This is especially true when the new behavior is harder to execute (like picking the right picture or remembering a word) than the old bad behavior, like screaming, hitting, or biting. If parents can both be consistent with any new demand, it will help the child overall—and the two of you can share the stress. Also, you will need to "pick your battles" and work on changing the most problematic behaviors first.

How to Address Communication Difficulties

Two key challenges arise in teaching children with an autism spectrum disorder to talk. Parents are key in overcoming both of these challenges. The first challenge is to teach your child what words mean. Learning that each person, place, thing, action, or experience has a name is the first big step that a child with autism must take. This is often accomplished by linking pictures and objects with specific vocabulary, usually starting with nouns, and usually starting with one example of each noun. Next, children are introduced to further examples of each "dog," "arm," "girl," "truck"—moving out from the first example. There is a substantial role here for parents—linking emerging language concepts to many examples to form the prototype of "dog," "arm," "girl," and "truck."

What does doing this look like? Say your child is learning "dog" and "cat." Make a trip to a pet store and look in at the kitties and puppies and ask what each is. Look at packaging of products and find more cats and dogs. Maybe some real dogs are walking around the store on leashes. When you read a story at night, find one that features dogs or cats and set things up so that identifying the cat or dog by name leads to an opportunity to turn a page or press a sound button or some other interesting, related action.

As a parent, it is your job to link those first examples of an object label to many examples that you and your child encounter every day. To do this, you need to know what vocabulary and concepts your child is learning from teachers and therapists. In a moment, we'll discuss how you can put that knowledge to use to best help your child.

Increasing Spontaneous Language Use

The second challenge is getting a child with an autism spectrum disorder to use the words he has. I often hear from parents who have had children in intensive therapies that their vocabulary now includes two or three hundred words—but only four or five are regularly used without being immediately modeled or otherwise prompted. Why is that?

There are many very different ideas out there about how to teach children with autism to talk. Behaviorists talk about teaching "verbal behavior." Verbal behavior can be divided into "tacting" (stating) and "manding" (requesting). Speech and language therapists tend to talk instead about language pragmatics and aspects like "proto-declarative" and "proto-imperative" speech, meaning—you guessed it—stating and requesting. You'll hear different terms that mean essentially the same thing. In any case, in this section we'll discuss your role in your child's language development, including working with speech and language therapists and teachers, as well as what you can do to ensure that the vocabulary your child learns in therapy and school is reinforced through natural practice opportunities you provide.

Speech and Language Therapy Cannot Be Done in a Black Box

Most children with autism spectrum disorders of any kind, as we discussed in the first part of this book, get speech and language therapy before anything else. The first time most parents think about a treatment "plan" they ask themselves—and anyone else who might have an opinion—"How much?" "How many times a week does he need speech therapy?"

Good questions, but not the most significant factor in how best to really help your child's communication abilities take root. Here are two analogies for what a speech therapist does and where you as a parent play a pivotal role in getting communication in gear:

First, think of what goes on in a speech therapy office as what it would be like for you to go to a foreign language class and spend hours with a teacher who was great at breaking things down just to the level that she knew you'd be able to follow. That's what a good speech therapist essentially does for a child with autism with a very limited ability to understand language. If you were to learn, say, Italian, you might be motivated by the idea that learning it would make it easier and more fun to communicate with all the relatives you were planning to meet on your trip to Italy. Your child, however, has much less of a basis for understanding why being a fluent speaker (even of a "first" language) might be so cool.

Let's take this analogy a step further: In learning a foreign language, your teacher might be great, but you would likely get much better once you spent a month with your family and really hit it off with them—immersion. Similarly, for your child to get the idea of why this language thing is so cool, he needs to use it outside speech therapy. This means that you need to be on top of what is happening and work with your child's therapist to make the lessons of speech therapy applicable outside the scaffolded learning environment of her office.

The second analogy: Speech and language therapy is like any other "rehab" (though it is actually *habilitative* rather than *rehabilitative*—your child is learning something he never knew, not relearning something he once knew). If you wrecked your back (as I did recently) and went to the physical therapist, the therapist might explain what's wrong, give you a short back massage for symptomatic relief, and very likely give you some exercises to do regularly at home. Which would be the best way for you to get better? Going three or four times a week for a massage and more demonstration exercises or actually following up and doing the assigned exercises three or four times a day? Obviously the latter. Speech therapy is essential the same deal. It is the constant exercise that produces improvements.

How Families Help

Exactly what role do you then take in this whole business of your child learning to talk? The first critical role for parents is in broadening the child's "linguistic prototypes" (as a developmental psycholinguist would say). A behaviorist would call it "generalizing" language. Interestingly, we know that in typically developing children a noun label is really a label for a prototype. From the time a baby starts to say a word like *nose*, the baby has the foundation for understanding that *nose* refers to a kind of template for something with two holes in the center of the face above the mouth. This understanding readily expands to include dog noses, clown noses, and even elephant "noses." As a parent, you are in the ideal position to help your child move from the one or two examples of each vocabulary word that the speech and language pathologist uses to other examples of those things. Autistic children do have more difficulty forming prototypes (partly because they can rigidly cling to the first example), so having other examples pointed out alongside the known examples (your "N-O-S-E" and doggy's "N-O-S-E") presents an ideal opportunity to promote generalization.

Augmentative Communication:
Do Pictures Keep Kids from Speaking?

Knowing which approach to take in teaching language is a tough one for many parents of children with autism who do not start to talk on time. Sign language has a certain cachet these days as it has come to be considered a baby "brain gym" activity for typically developing eight- to twelve-month-olds. If your child is not talking, is that the route you should go? If your child does not point, automatically look where you look, or catch your eye and then look at an object of interest, he probably does not have the right prerequisites for sign language. Sign language is just a bigger, better, more formal system of nonverbal communication. If nonverbal communication is an area of weakness for your child, it's not likely to be a good way to compensate for not understanding word meanings if that is another area of weakness. So what should you do?

You and your child's speech and language therapist need to work this out. Different therapists do different things with different children, and most combine approaches. You are likely to see three different approaches: In the first, the child and the therapist spend lots of time playing together, rolling cars and trains, feeding dolls, and using other natural contexts that can promote receptive language ("Give the dolly his bottle!") as well as reciprocity ("Your turn!" "My turn!"). In the second approach, work focuses on getting the child to practice speech sounds and/or words, articulating more clearly, and using longer utterances if the child is already speaking. In the third approach, the child is introduced to "augmentative communication"—some sort of picture communication.

Many speech and language therapists and teachers use a method called the PECS (Picture Exchange Communication System), which is based mainly on little black-and-white or colored line drawings that the child "exchanges" for the object represented. Many parents don't like this because it seems very unnatural, with rows of small one-inch-square picture cards attached to a binder page with Velcro, row after row, page after page. It seems like giving a visitor to a foreign country a pictorial phrase book and expecting the natives of this country to stand around while you thumb through your book, snatching pictures to show that "Me" and "My husband" want to take the "Bus" and go to the "Train station." It would be very rote, but if the natives of this country were accustomed to visitors doing this sort of thing, it might work. In school, PECS can become what the child is accustomed to doing, but few parents fully implement this system at home. PECS certainly can and does work in special education classes, but what about in the real world? Specifically, what about at home? What parents need is a system that is practical, addresses specific language learning problems *their* child is having, motivates the child to want to communicate more and/or more appropriately, and encourages spoken language over just using pictures.

How Families Help

The modified system I always recommend to parents to use at home is VIA (visual interaction augmentation), which is more fully described in my book *Helping Children with Autism Learn* (see Resources at the end of this book). VIA is based more on how typically developing children learn to talk—incorporating behavioral principles and developmentally based content. Basically, you use real photos of specific real things (like a picture of a small green box of Tree Top apple juice—if this is the juice your child drinks), not generic line drawings (like a glass that is yellowy-orange below the fill line). The child with autism thinks in "pictures"—but the pictures are not stick figures and line drawings; they are in living color. You can put these pictures around the house—wherever the pictured items are located. (You do this with lots of Velcro and lots of copies of each photo for when the picture falls behind the sofa, gets eaten by the dog, or is snatched by a baby sibling.) Your job is to use these pictures to create natural opportunities to get your child to practice communicating—whenever he wants something.

The idea is to show your child opportunities where a picture, a word approximation clarified by a picture, or a word prompted by a picture is the key to getting activities, foods, toys, and choices that he wants. When the child wants something he sees in a picture, he is taught to bring you the picture. You are taught to hold the picture to your face, point between the picture, the child, and your eyes, and as soon as you think the child "sees" that you know what he wants (say, by looking between your eyes and the picture), you fulfill his request. This way, you are naturally teaching your child to "read" your eyes, follow a point, and "read" your face.

This also gives you an opportunity to say the word your child is trying to learn. Say it many times. Say it in context. This will link the word to its meaning as well as promoting the generalization that's so important. The speech and language therapist does not live at your house. She can't do this. Only *you* can make spontaneous instrumental communication something that your child comes to see as valuable.

Can Computers Teach Communication?

Another way parents often try to facilitate their child's development is through the use of computers. Many children with autism really gravitate to computers because they are basically nonsocial interaction partners. Computers quickly become completely predictable—and certainly do not eschew repetitiveness. For a child with autism, life with a computer can be quite copacetic as there are none of those hard-to-understand, unpredictable social cues. For parents of children with autism, however, computers are a mixed bag. On one hand, the American Academy of Pediatrics recommends no more than ninety minutes of "screen time" (live TV, recorded videos, video games plus computers) each day for all school-age children and *no* screen time for children under two. (It would be safe to guess that no one from the Media Committee of the American Academy of Pediatrics is on the board of the companies that produce Baby Einstein or Baby Mozart videos, or *Teletubbies*.) On the other hand, parents see for themselves that the child can pay attention for much longer to anything on the computer than anything "live" and that he has learned letters, numbers, shapes, colors, and animal names from the computer. But sometimes the computer has become so valued by the child that the most predictable meltdowns come when it must be turned off. How do you strike a balance?

The first rule is to limit time. A half hour at one sitting is plenty if we are talking about educational games. Some computer games are educational when they dovetail with other things your child is learning, especially when the computer reinforces concepts that have already been introduced by live human beings. However, just because a piece of software is *called* "educational" doesn't mean that it is. The real world takes place beyond the screen.

The second rule is to limit the amount of time that computer use is a solitary activity. Is there a sibling who can play along or "teach"? Can you watch? Many times parents who use the computer as an electronic binky do not realize that either the child is not playing meaningfully or that he is playing repetitively.

For certain children, just getting a reaction on the screen to your action with the mouse is enough, and minutes can pass clicking randomly and going with the resulting flow. If the child does not yet "get" the one-to-one correspondence of the mouse action and the screen, it might be good to consider a touch screen instead. (With a touch screen the child responds by directly touching the thing he would otherwise click.) For the youngest children, in any case, this is a good first step in using the computer to help develop cause-and-effect reasoning.

Left on their own at a computer, other children glom on to a single subroutine—and always choose the "cow" subroutine though the video barnyard is inhabited by a whole menagerie. By sitting with the child, you can present a choice: meet a new animal or choose another game *or* turn off the computer altogether.

This brings us to the third rule: Manage the tendency to get obsessed with the computer. Get a "Time Timer" (available from special education catalogs) or any countdown timer from RadioShack. Set the time your child is allowed to use the computer. (On a Time Timer, the portion of a sixty-minute clock face designating the allocated amount of time shows as a red wedge, getting thinner until it finally disappears.) Remind your child when the time is almost up. When time *is* up, count to three and be prepared to turn off the screen if the child has not started to "exit." Yes, this may provoke a tantrum, but this is an opportunity to show your child that there is structure and there are rules to be followed at home just like at school, and that you are in charge. Be ready to redirect your child to something else acceptable if not preferred. The limit needs to be firm, however. If you are firm and consistent, you can expect a struggle at first, but eventual acceptance of the limit. Of course, this works best if everyone in the house can be on the same page with limiting computer use.

In addition to all these guidelines, know that there are special software programs designed to help language comprehension in a child, like most language-delayed autistic children, who are visual more than auditory learners. These include things like TeachTown, Laureate Learning Systems products, and Earobics. These are not your CompUSA kiddy-software packages, but professional products that cost some real money and have subprograms tailored for different levels of language comprehension, expression, and speed of auditory processing. If computers do seem like a good learning modality for your child, ask your speech and language pathologist, special day class teacher, or home program supervisor to help you investigate them and make some recommendations about specific programs your child is ready for.

Developing Play

The next big area where parents can make a difference for their children is in the area of play development. The term *play* really has two major dimensions. The first is play with toys and games; the second is play with other children—meaning play can enhance communication as well as social skills, thus addressing two of the major barriers to learning. Why is play important?

Play as Language Practice

Play is the way children practice language. As children play, they repeat words and phrases they've heard in the scenarios they reenact. This reinforces the meaning of words. This can be something as simple as making backing-up "beeps" while rolling a truck backward to more complex scenes wherein one doll who has bitten another is told "I don't like to see inappropriate behavior." Parents of children with autism spectrum disorders can be too sensitized to hearing their children use whole phrases like "I don't like to see inappropriate behavior," worrying that the child is being echolalic and that echolalia is all bad. Echolalia is not all bad, and in fact, echolalia is an expected strategy in early language development as children move from one- and two-word phrases to larger, more complex statements. What we would call *functional delayed echolalia* in a child with autism is, more importantly, a sign that the child is trying to use a strong auditory memory to power through a sentence's meaning when she can't readily recall meaning from more nuanced vocabulary or grammar.

The child's doing this tells us she's hearing fast enough (doesn't have auditory processing delays) but may have central processing problems in the part of the brain where a whole phrase should be taken apart and each word recognized and stored separately. This is the place where you can step in and help your child by breaking down the language: "Oh, is 'inappropriate' bad or good?" "Bad?" "Oh, biting is bad! Bad dolly!" Children who echo large pieces of video scripts can be helped by playing along with the video so their Nemo can do and say what the video Nemo does at the same time. When you play with your child using his "TV talk" as a script, you bring word meaning and action closer together.

Restating an echoed utterance in simpler words can help your child in the same way. If your child has said something, it means something for him. Simply ignoring echolalia or discouraging it (as if it were an "inappropriate behavior") bypasses the opportunity to make your child's communicative attempt successful and thereby rewarding. If you help echolalia become meaningful, your child will try to talk more, rather than less. Ignoring echolalia without helping your child revise it says to him, "Don't talk to me; it doesn't help me understand you." Not surprisingly, parents who have been told to ignore echolalic speech end up being concerned that their child doesn't have much spontaneous language. If you can, instead, rephrase what the echolalia means and respond to that, you are giving your child a reason to try to get through to you with his words in the future.

Play as "Thinking" Practice

Play is also important because it is the forerunner of abstract thinking. When a child constructs a scene where one doll is reprimanded for biting another, the child scripting that scene has done a great job of stripping the action down to the key essentials. What the biting doll is wearing, what color doll it is, and whether the other doll is a cute Teletubbie or a scary Batman falls away in the context of "biting" as the topic. Mastering this type of play later maps onto the ability to do something like a math word problem: "Two boys raked leaves for two hours and earned two dollars an hour. How much money did they get?" Leaves are not important, nor are the rakes. We certainly know that many children with autism are much better computationally with math than at word problems with much simpler mathematical operations. This is one reason why. Play that is silly, even absurd, and stripped down to essentials, is not a waste of time compared to doing math fact drills. Both are needed for later success. Let the teachers do the math fact drills. Your job is to play with your child in a way that breeds flexible abstract thinking. This can be something as silly and stupid as having Batman bite the Teletubbie back and then telling Batman, "I don't like to see inappropriate behavior" and repeating this script ten more times with five or six other favorite characters.

Many parents limit toy play time for two reasons: First, it takes time from "work"—such as tabletop tasks. Second, the play seems repetitive and meaningless and therefore like mental downtime. Remember that all work and no play makes Jack a dull boy. Even if Jack has autism. However, you are quite right in not wanting to see highly repetitive play. Here is another place where parents can help.

How Families Help

Play is supposed to be fun. One of the reasons play is fun is that the child decides for herself what she will do. If you decide to leave work early on a Friday and check out a sale at your favorite clothing store, you might say you were going to "*play* hooky" and go have some fun. A big source of fun is that you have *chosen* what to do. Autistic children like to have fun and choose what to do too. The problem comes in only when the choice is repetitive (playing the same three minutes of video over and over) or is pretty infantile (spinning something and getting excited as a nine-month-old might). The challenge in getting a child with autism to play "better" is to decrease the repetitiveness that feeds into mental downtime and move forward the developmental level of the play—moving the child closer to activities and interests shared by others his age.

How do you do this? For starters, you need to play with things your child likes. This means if your child is obsessed with Thomas the

Tank Engine, you don't take it away but rather give him a choice: The choice is playing with Thomas in a slightly new way (that you support) or *not* playing with Thomas.

What does this look like? It looks like what these days is getting called Floortime/DIR or RDI, described in Chapter 7. These packaged approaches are derivatives of the type of child play therapy that child psychiatrists, child psychologists, and child social workers all learn. While you can attend a training session on how to use one of these methods, don't feel you have to in order to help your child become a better player. I certainly know many parents who have gotten organized, galvanized, and even certified by attending a DIR or RDI workshop. You definitely need all the support you can get, so if it's appealing, consider doing something like this. The principles of play, however, are simple. It's nice to have a workbook (like with RDI)—but you don't need a workbook to play with your child in a manner that will support his developmental goals.

The most basic principle of motivating play for the child with autism is to identify things your child likes to play with. Why does she like them? Because they spin? Because they light up? Because they are balls? If your child has a preferred category of toys, she probably already has a lot of them. Let's say, for argument's sake, that your two-and-a-half-year-old has two hundred different kinds of balls—because she really likes balls. Put some of them away to keep them "fresh." Okay. What does she like to do with balls? If she can throw them, can she kick them? Can she roll them to someone else? Can she throw one and get it back from a retriever-like dog? Think of variations on this theme. Think of how you can insinuate yourself into these variations. If your child loves putting Thomas around the track *very* repetitively, and has made it clear to you that you have no real role in this, start with putting your hand over the track as Thomas approaches and say "Stop!" and then instantly remove your hand and say "Go!" as described in the last chapter—and let your child continue. After "Stop!" "Go!" becomes a routine, make it a longer stop and see if your child will tolerate your bending over and getting in his face before you smile and announce "Go!" If this becomes a routine, you can expect your child to start looking for that smile to see if it's a "Go!" When you get to that point, your activity looks a bit like interactive play. For some kids, this can be slow going. For some kids, there is more resistance than for others. Time the duration and intensity of your bouts of play to match what the child can take. The play activity itself should continue to be fun (a preferred choice), but the fun should wear off on the variation on the theme so that you have successfully broadened your child's play horizons.

Child Play-Coaching Models

But, you say, when am I supposed to do this play thing? What about my job, my other kids, my spouse, and my life as a carpool operator? The answer is other children. Historically, other children have been the source of inculcating and transmitting play. I will never forget this fact, because many years ago at my PhD orals at Stanford, I was asked, rather out of the blue, what the average age of a caregiver in the Third World was. I did not know. I think I guessed twelve or thirteen. The answer is eight. An eight-year-old girl has a lot more energy for playing with your child than you do. An eight-year-old girl who is empowered to be a bit bossy ("It's okay if you're bossy, because sometimes he just wants to do it his way . . . ") can be very helpful. The idea is to find a child who's insistent but not mean—a "big sister" or "little mother" type. I would consider going so far as to offer such a child a couple bucks an hour to come over and "be in charge" of your child for an hour at a time. You want the kind of insistent, intrusive child whose mother is *glad* to have her come to your house for a while. At first you'll need to supervise this play a bit, but the idea is for it to take on a life of its own without your micromanagement.

Teen Tutors

Another child-coaching model is the teen tutor. A teen tutor is a high school student who really likes kids and is happy to earn babysitting money from 3 to 5 on Tuesdays and Thursdays instead of giving up four hours on a Saturday night. You might initially spend a little time telling her what your child likes and doesn't like, can do and cannot do, and sticking around long enough to see if they gibe. (This is basically what you might do briefly with any new potential babysitter.) With a teen, you can explain a little about autism, how you don't want him to just do the same thing over and over, that you want him to use his words (or picture choices), no TV, videos, or computer games—and then let her loose. Outdoor activities that burn more steam than you have at the end of the day (like twenty minutes on a trampoline) are great choices.

Teen tutors are also my first choice as facilitators of play dates. Yes, you can facilitate a play date. A trained ABA tutor can facilitate a play date. But you want play to be fun, right? While many ABA agencies include play date supervision as part of what they do, you might negotiate to have the ABA tutor model/train a teen tutor in running a play date—and then back off. The teen is going to be younger—and probably more open-ended in play. It also can be hard for both your child and an ABA tutor to switch from teacher–student to player–playmate roles.

Siblings

The only simple caveat about peer and teen tutors is to limit the use of siblings. Cousins, fine. Siblings—not so much. Siblings have enough on their plates without having to feel they are the only ones, or the best ones, to get their autistic brother or sister to talk or play. If your ideal peer tutor would be a child the same age as your older daughter or son, you need a slightly different solution. You can't expect an eight-year-old to come to the house of another eight-year-old and have them not play together, or even together with the younger sibling with autism. In this case, setting up play outside the home (which we will discuss in a minute) might work out more smoothly.

Developing Friendships

Play coaching from bossy older children and teens is a fine way to demonstrate to your child the joys of social interaction. Of most concern to many parents, however, is the fact that their child has little or no interest in other children. For many moms, lack of interest in peer affiliation (say, in a Mommy and Me play group) is the first real worry.

Play with other children *is* important because the affiliative drive that underpins it underlies important avenues for learning: Seeing another child use a familiar toy in a new way, or a new toy in a familiar way, should trigger a little snapshot in your child's head—which can later be used as a blueprint for your child to try to do the same thing. Affiliative drive is also what later motivates whole groups of children to behave according to norms set in school.

Affiliative drive is the innate desire to do like, be like, be with, and be accepted and liked by others. It may seem to you that your child was taking a nap when everyone else lined up to get their "affiliative drive." How can we stimulate the development of this interest in learning from others?

Developmental Inclusion

Different formal and informal approaches have been taken. What you as a parent need to know are some of the basic principles of these. You can also follow a few guidelines as you look for programs and placements you hope will help your child become more social. The first is that you need to appraise your child's play developmentally. Say your child with an autism spectrum disorder is four years old. When he's put in a sandbox at the park, his specialty is "dump and pour." You notice that everyone else in the sandbox doing "dump and pour" is about two. The other four-year-olds are copying each other doing different kinds of belly-flops down the slide. What do you do if you want your child to play with others? Take him over to the slide, interrupt the four-year-olds, and insist they give your son a turn, even though he is screaming and refusing to climb the ladder? No, he's not a four-year-old player yet. Let's help him be a two-year-old player and social (as social goes for two-year-olds) as a first step. Maybe you could help him take turns with a two-year-old who is busy filling a big pit. All you're going for is some sense of mutuality—as that's about it for interaction among two-year-olds. If you can foster that awareness on the part of your child, you can hope for more spontaneous awareness, and perhaps even some deferred imitation of other two-year-old activities in the future. He's not going to imitate other kids belly-flopping down the slide at the get-go—that's still too complex to combine with emerging observation and imitation skills.

Another choice is to encourage your child to play with kids who are five or six or older—who in a free-play setting will readily simplify their own play overtures to match a playmate. This can be hard at a park—where the five- or six-year-old may have many choices—but can work well in your living room if a friend has come over with her six-year-old and there are only the two of them.

Why am I saying that your preschool-age child with an autism spectrum disorder should have either younger or older playmates? What about preschool inclusion? Isn't playing with other kids his own age better? Yes—that's certainly the goal. To get there, however, play with either developmentally equivalent (younger) children or (older) children developmentally able to scaffold social interaction offers the best probability of a connection. Other two-, three-, four-, and sometimes five-year-olds lack the skill, interest, and patience to play with someone developmentally different from themselves. Developmentally, by the time children are five or six, they are usually capable mentally of doing essentially what adults do—which is to bend down, get attention, adjust speech, adjust interests, get physical, etc.—all to rope in the interest of the child who does not yet seem to connect with them.

Peer Experiences: Where?

A first peer integration experience may work best in a mixed-age family day care program or other after-school site. A neighborhood recreation center or pool or beach or park is likely to afford such opportunity as well. I particularly like family day care for this purpose, because the setting is small, the play area contained, and the peer group stable—unlike at a public facility.

This does not mean there is no role for inclusion in a typical preschool for your child. For children who already have some ability to follow a routine, observe, and imitate, there definitely are advantages of preschool inclusion. If your child is, however, two or three years younger developmentally than the other preschoolers, it may be hard for the goings-on to be the kinds of things he is going to want to observe or imitate. When kids like this are placed in typical preschools anyway, they need full-time shadow aides, who usually end up either providing a program-within-a-program or simply removing your child when he can no longer tolerate being quiet and holding still during an activity that is still way above him developmentally. (Would you want to sit in a physics class if you hated both math and science classes in school? Put yourself in your child's shoes for this one.)

One-to-one shadowing is likely to be needed, at least initially, for any child with an autism spectrum disorder who is joining in with typical peers for the first time. How much shadowing is needed depends on where your child is developmentally, where the peers are developmentally, and how large and structured the group activity is. Shadows should be just that—shadows, staying as much in the background as possible and not serving as personal handmaidens. If you are in the position of identifying a shadow for your child—say for a private preschool—you should be looking for someone sensitive to how much your child can do on her own and where she needs supports. A shadow should also be able to pick out altruistic play partners for your child and make play with your child inviting, by creating a center of action in which your child is naturally included.

From Knowing What You Want to Working Successfully with Treatment Providers

This chapter has explained how you can do things or set things up so that specific teaching strategies as well as everyday activities foster language, play, and overall development. Once you are at this point— understanding how your child learns, understanding what different comprehensive programs should be able to do, understanding all the "wraparound" pieces that you and others will need to support so that your child is motivated, attentive, and ready to participate in instruction—you are ready: You're ready to face an IFSP or IEP team with a great deal of information about different treatment strategies, as well as about how your child in particular is likely to learn best.

In the next chapter, armed with what you now know about what your child needs, we will take on navigating the laws and practices that govern publicly funded special education services for your child.

PART IV

On the Road

GETTING OUT THERE
TO GET WHAT YOU NEED

Up until this point in this book, you've been listening to one voice: my voice. I may understand many things about autism, but certainly much less about the laws that regulate the services you will need for your child. These days parents are well served to know their legal rights with respect to their child's treatments as well. Therefore, in the next chapter, I have invited a prominent special education attorney, Kathryn Dobel, to walk you through this often challenging part of the maze that leads to getting the best possible treatment for your child.

Then, once you have arrived at the best treatment plan that your child is entitled to by law, you'll be ready to dive in as a collaborative member of your child's treatment team. Chapter 10 will help you move through day-to-day dealings with the therapists, agencies, teachers, and schools who provide your child with help.

NINE

Navigating
the Legal Byways

ENTITLEMENTS THAT FOSTER LEARNING

Kathryn E. Dobel

Thanks and my deepest appreciation to Kathryn E. Dobel, an attorney specializing in law surrounding the special education of children with autism, for writing this chapter. Ms. Dobel has been representing families of children with autism for over twenty-five years. She prevailed in the first case in both California and the United States on behalf of parents seeking reimbursement for costs of treatment for early intervention at UCLA's Early Autism Project. Subsequently, she has represented families throughout the western United States. She is a founding board member and past chair of the Council of Parent Attorneys and Advocates (COPAA), a national organization founded with the purpose of education and protection of the rights of students with disabilities; co-chair of the California Association for Parent–Child Advocacy (CAPCA); and the Northern California site instructor for the Special Education Advocacy Training Project, a project of the Office of Special Education and Rehabilitative Services (OSERS), cosponsored by the University of Southern California University Center for Excellence in Developmental Disabilities (USC UCEDD) and COPAA. The Resources section of this book tells you how to get a more detailed version of this chapter that includes extensive citations and case references that might be of help to an advocate or lawyer representing you and your child with autism in a special education matter.

A big part of arriving at the best possible treatment for a child with autism is knowing your child's rights under the law and how that law translates into the provision of services through the schools and other avenues. Children diagnosed with autism spectrum disorders qualify for special education and related services according to the federal Individuals with Disabilities Education Improvement Act of 2004 (IDEA). The purpose of the IDEA is "to ensure that all children with disabilities have available to them a free appropriate public education that emphasizes special education and related services designed to meet their unique needs and prepare them for further education, employment and independent living" and "to ensure that the rights of children with disabilities and parents of such children are protected."

The IDEA is the most recent in a series of statutes ensuring the educational rights of students with disabilities, the first of which was enacted in 1975. In the IDEA of 2004, Congress sets forth fourteen important findings related to educating children with disabilities, including the following:

(1) Disability is part of the human experience and in no way diminishes the right of individuals to participate in, or contribute to society. Improving educational results for children with disabilities is an essential element of our national policy of ensuring equality of opportunity, full participation, independent living and economic self-sufficiency for individuals with disabilities. . . .

(5) Almost 30 years of research and experience has demonstrated that the education of children with disabilities can be made more effective by

(A) having high expectations for such children and ensuring their access to the general education curriculum in the regular classroom, to the maximum extent possible, in order to (i) meet developmental goals and, to the maximum extent possible, the challenging expectations that have been established for all children; (ii) be prepared to lead productive and independent adult lives, to the maximum extent possible.

(B) strengthening the role and responsibility of parents and ensuring that families of such children have meaningful opportunities to participate in the education of their children at school and at home. . . .

(E) . . . improve the academic achievement and functional performance of children with disabilities, including the use of scientifically based instructional practices, to the maximum extent possible . . . And . . .

(H) supporting the development and use of technology, including assistive technology devices and assistive technology services, to maximize accessibility for children with disabilities.

The core of the IDEA is the individualized education program (IEP)—called the individualized family service plan (IFSP) for children from birth through age three—which is the critical link between your child with disabilities and the special education and related services the child needs. Special education is defined by the federal law as "specially designed instruction at no cost to parents, to meet the unique needs of a child with a disability, including instruction conducted in the classroom, in the home, in hospitals and institutions, and in other settings." Your state must enact a statute or statutes providing for the protections and procedures that the federal law mandates, and it can require the school districts in your state to provide more, but not less, than the federal law demands for educating children with disabilities. You will need to check with local resources for guidance on whether your state provides for more than the federal law requires.

As explained earlier in this book, the IEP is the written program developed for your child that outlines his current special education needs, goals for the next twelve months to address these needs, and programs, placements, and services to implement the program developed by the IEP team. The IEP is also a management tool designed to assure that the program is appropriate for the child's individual education needs and is actually delivered and monitored. This means the special education program laid out in the IEP must focus on *your* child's individual needs and not on an entire class of children.

Progress toward reaching the goals specified in the IEP will be measured at least annually. (The IDEA of 2004 also allows states to give parents and school districts the option of developing a comprehensive multiyear IEP, designed to coincide with the natural transition points for the child, such as preschool to elementary grades, elementary grades to middle or junior high school grades, from secondary school grades to postsecondary activities, but in no case covering a period longer than three years. For autism, however, this option rarely makes sense.)

The vision set forth by the IDEA and the purpose of the IEP seem pretty straightforward, but in practice when you seek special education services for your child you're entering a maze that can be tricky to navigate. The navigational challenge starts with the fact that in no other field are there as many acronyms and abbreviations as in special education. As the blueprint for your child's special education, the IEP is the acronym most important to your family. The goal of this chapter is to help you play your role as an effective equal participant (among other participants dictated by the law, listed in the sidebar on page 209) in the development of your child's IEP by knowing:

- What your child is entitled to
- How to prepare for IEP meetings
- How to contribute to the program being developed
- And how to follow up once a plan is proposed.

Underlying this process is another critical acronym: Your child is legally entitled by law to a *free and appropriate public education* (FAPE). This concept is both tremendously empowering in what it makes available to your child and potentially frustrating, as the meaning of "appropriate" is subjective—and subject to legal and public policy debate. I'll explain how the term *appropriate* may be interpreted legally for your child with autism as of early 2007, but keep in mind that what is appropriate for one child is not the same as what will be appropriate for another, even if they both have autism. In addition, the legal concept of an appropriate public education will continue to evolve. If you're working with a lay advocate or special education attorney, he or she should be able to walk you through how the current law itself has laid out what an IEP must include in the service of providing FAPE. An advocate is a nonattorney who has pursued special training in education law. There are some excellent, well-trained advocates in special education law, and such an advocate can be one cost-effective approach to getting support through the IEP process. Some advocates are parents of children with autism who may have an ax to grind because of difficulties encountered in planning for their own child. Be a little more cautious in selecting such an advocate if you sense his or her approach to the school is more personal than professional. An attorney who specializes in special education advocacy may be your best guarantee of knowledgeable support. Try to find an attorney who has a track record of being able to settle with schools, not just suing them— or you may ultimately find yourself wondering how much of his new Mercedes *you* paid for. Many locales have Protection and Advocacy (PAI) organizations that provide pro bono or sliding-scale legal assis-

---

Who's on the IEP Team?

The IDEA requires that the following people be members of the IEP team:

- You, the parents of the child with an autism spectrum disorder
- At least one of the child's regular education teachers if the child is, or may be, participating in the regular education environment
- At least one special education teacher or, where appropriate, not less than one autism specialist or service provider, such as the behavioral specialist
- A representative of the local educational agency who:
  a. Is qualified to provide, or supervise the provision of, specially designed instruction to meet the unique needs of children with disabilities
  b. Is knowledgeable about the general education curriculum and
  c. Is knowledgeable about the availability of resources of the local educational agency
- An individual who can interpret the instructional implications of evaluation results (such as a school psychologist or other person who tested your child as eligible for special education services)
- Other individuals who have knowledge or special expertise regarding the child, including related services personnel as appropriate—at the discretion of the parent or the agency
- The child, whenever appropriate, such as a teen with high-functioning autism or Asperger syndrome who should be part of his transition out of school-related services

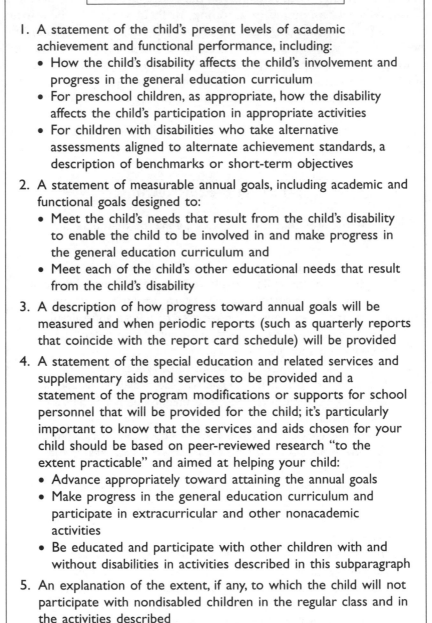

What the IEP Includes

1. A statement of the child's present levels of academic achievement and functional performance, including:
   - How the child's disability affects the child's involvement and progress in the general education curriculum
   - For preschool children, as appropriate, how the disability affects the child's participation in appropriate activities
   - For children with disabilities who take alternative assessments aligned to alternate achievement standards, a description of benchmarks or short-term objectives

2. A statement of measurable annual goals, including academic and functional goals designed to:
   - Meet the child's needs that result from the child's disability to enable the child to be involved in and make progress in the general education curriculum and
   - Meet each of the child's other educational needs that result from the child's disability

3. A description of how progress toward annual goals will be measured and when periodic reports (such as quarterly reports that coincide with the report card schedule) will be provided

4. A statement of the special education and related services and supplementary aids and services to be provided and a statement of the program modifications or supports for school personnel that will be provided for the child; it's particularly important to know that the services and aids chosen for your child should be based on peer-reviewed research "to the extent practicable" and aimed at helping your child:
   - Advance appropriately toward attaining the annual goals
   - Make progress in the general education curriculum and participate in extracurricular and other nonacademic activities
   - Be educated and participate with other children with and without disabilities in activities described in this subparagraph

5. An explanation of the extent, if any, to which the child will not participate with nondisabled children in the regular class and in the activities described

6. A statement of any accommodations deemed necessary to

measure the child's academic achievement and functioning on state- and districtwide assessments and an explanation of why alternative assessments should be made instead if that is considered appropriate

7. The projected date for starting the services and modifications and how often, where, and for how long they will take place

8. Provisions for postsecondary goals and transition services, starting with the first IEP in effect when the child is sixteen, and a statement of any rights that transfer to the child upon majority, made at least one year before majority

tance. In any case, don't feel that legal representation at an IEP meeting is necessarily where you should start. Schools see initial inclusion of your legal representative as a statement of distrust of the school—which is no way to start a long-term relationship. However, if you feel you would be on more solid ground with representation, then, by all means, seek out an advocate or attorney.

How to Get Started: Preparing for the IEP Meeting

Contact your local educational agency to request an IEP (or IFSP if your child is less than three years old) as soon as an assessment of your child has raised developmental concerns (see Chapters 1–3). Your child does not need a diagnosis to be eligible for help. The public agency may do some assessment of their own—to figure out where the most appropriate services may be. You should get started with the IEP process as soon as you can. If you get further assessments that suggest different or additional services or teaching strategies, you can always ask for another IEP meeting. Immediately begin preparation for the IEP meeting as if you were drawing a blueprint for your house with an architect.

Your school district will send you a written notice of the upcoming IEP meeting. Carefully read the list of people scheduled to attend the meeting and ask the school district to invite anyone not on the list who you think is important to the team making decisions about your child—or invite them yourself. Let the person organizing your meeting know who you will be bringing. Make sure from the outset that sufficient time is allotted for the meeting. A detailed IEP may take from a few to many hours to prepare. Don't let the school staff schedule only one hour and then have to convene additional meetings to complete the IEP. This will make you weary, and wary of the school district's motivations as well as its expertise.

How do you begin to plan for this important meeting? Start with the necessary assessments of your child.

Gathering the Appropriate Assessments before the IEP Meeting

Obviously, before an appropriate remedial program can be designed, you have to know what your child's disability is, which requires a thorough evaluation. Unfortunately, school district evaluations for preschool children with autism spectrum disorders are often limited by time, the experience of the evaluator, and the scope of the assessment. Rarely do school assessors provide a specific diagnosis, and the diagnostic categories that educators use are different from those used by psychologists and psychiatrists. Even the category of "autism" is different, often more broadly defined by a school authority than by a doctor. In addition to the school-based assessments being possibly more limited in scope, a child who hasn't yet had early intensive behavioral treatment may not be amenable to cooperating with tests given by the average school psychologist or special education teacher using standardized instruments. This means the most important initial data gathered by the school team most likely will come from you.

The Importance of Parent Reports and Independent Assessments

A major goal of the assessments is not just to determine what your child's disability is but also to measure specifically how your child performs academically and functions in general. Parents usually know their children best, so you'll want to make sure the written reports you receive from the school's evaluators accurately reflect what you told the school district team during the assessment interview.

But good assessment data from standardized test instruments are also critical to planning your child's IEP, so if your child can be assessed in a meaningful way, be sure those are employed. The data from these assessments, as well as day-to-day functioning skills you observe, will determine the baseline for your child's academic achievement and functional performance. All future progress will be measured from this baseline to make sure the plan is effective for your child, so clearly, getting an accurate baseline picture of your child's abilities is essential.

If at all possible, also provide the school assessment team with information from a thorough diagnostic assessment you've gotten on your own. Ideally, these independent evaluators should present assessments and recommendations to the IEP team, but in practical terms that may be possible only through video or teleconferencing since it can be hard to coordinate the schedules of so many individuals for the IEP meeting.

It's best to get an independent evaluation from an autism spectrum disorder expert experienced in designing and monitoring progress from IEPs. Not all autism diagnosticians have much contact with the educational system, so if you're looking for a diagnostician who can write recommendations that will make sense to educators, ascertain that as part of selecting an evaluator, as discussed in Chapter 5. Local chapters of the Autism Society of America and Families for Effective Autism Treatment (FEAT), as well as other organizations in your area (see the Resources at the end of this book), should have referral lists for professionals who perform thorough evaluations for autism spectrum disorders.

If the school assessment hasn't provided adequate information regarding diagnosis insofar as it bears on placement, or, most important, on present levels of performance, among other things, you have the right to seek reimbursement from the school district for this independent assessment. Whether the school district will agree to reimburse you without dispute is questionable, but the data from the outside evaluation must be included in the IEP discussion no matter who pays for the evaluation.

Why You Need to Get Reports before the IEP Meeting

You may and should request copies of the written reports from the school assessment team before the IEP meeting. I recommend that you receive the reports at least five days prior to the IEP meeting so you'll have some idea how the school staff views your child and whether an independent evaluation is warranted. You don't want to see the reports for the first time at the meeting; you'll need time to read them carefully before being able to participate in a discussion about these evaluations at the IEP. If the reports aren't available until the day of the meeting, you'll have to decide whether to request a postponement.

Unfortunately, if reading the school team's reports indicates the need for an independent evaluation, there can be a wait for an appointment with an experienced expert. So what do you do if the independent evaluation won't be done until after the date scheduled for the IEP meeting? While you can request a postponement of the meeting, that's not always a good idea if it means your child will end up without any adequate program or services for an extended period of time. So you could choose to go ahead with the meeting, while exercising your right not to agree to the ultimate IEP wording until you believe the plan accurately reflects your child's identified needs.

Writing Your Own Statement of Your Child's Current Abilities

Before the IEP meeting, create your own detailed written statement of how you see your child in all developmental domains across settings (at home, in the community, and at school or in other group-based programs), including behavioral, cognitive, social/play, emotional, speech/ language and communication, fine and gross motor, preacademic and academic, and self-help domains. Be sure to take it to the IEP meeting, but it's even better if you can share it, along with any outside evaluations you've obtained, in advance with the school district IEP team members so the meeting won't be delayed by the reading of your reports for the first time. In fact, you might consider writing this statement when you first inquire about an IEP, because your report could help all the evaluators who will be assessing your child plan which assessment instruments to use.

At the Meeting: Setting Goals and Objectives

The IEP team will discuss your child's present levels of academic achievement and functional performance based on the evaluations; observations of your child at home, at school, and in the community; and data collection. This baseline information will be recorded on the Present Levels of Academic Achievement and Functional Performance (PLOAA and FP) documentation. Here's a good example of how specific the present-level data should look for one behavioral area:

> *Present Level* (Jargoning): Student verbalizes phrases that serve no apparent functional purpose. These phrases are usually dialogue from familiar movies and storybooks. Student exhibits this behavior when a demand is

placed on him and while playing alone. In response to a demand during work sessions, student exhibits this behavior 1 of 10 probed occasions. It occurs when student is not engaged on another 5 of 10 probed occasions.

The first goal of the team's discussion is to emerge with a clear picture of your child's strengths and weaknesses for the purposes of IEP planning. From the summary of strengths and weaknesses, the team will formulate semiannual or annual goals and short-term objectives or benchmarks. Anyone who has attended a business meeting, where goals are determined and responsibilities are assigned, will readily understand this process. Be forewarned, however, that in the school setting you may not find this process as well organized as it can be at the office, depending on the skill level and expertise of the school staff developing the IEP. You may be most comfortable in corporate culture and readily understand its advantages in negotiation, but the culture of education is more like a merchants' association for very small businesses—with each classroom its own small business. This is the perspective that virtually all school-based IEP team members have to bring with them to the IEP meeting.

Not Too High or Too Low

The goals and objectives for your child must be measurable and based on reasonable expectations of progress given an appropriate program. We'll get further into what is "reasonable" and "appropriate" later, but for now, understand this is something of a balancing act. First, the goals and objectives are not contractual obligations. But beware of goals that are either too low or too high. Goals that are not well thought out or realistic will only frustrate everyone and could send the IEP team on a wild goose chase for ways to revise the services to make the goals achievable, when it's actually the goals that need rethinking. I am usually more concerned, however, about having the bar set *too low*. The federal law cautions IEP teams against "low expectations," and when the goals set for your child are too low, the IEP may unnecessarily limit expectations—and therefore opportunities—for significant developmental changes. So ask yourself whether the goals set for your child gibe with what you know of your child's autism-specific learning disabilities (ALDs) and autistic learning styles (ALSs).

At this point in the development of the IEP it would be premature to make definitive judgments about curriculum content and methods, but you should still be alert to whether what is beginning to take shape *seems* likely to permit your child to make sequential developmental gains. You've taken a very close look at your child's strengths and weaknesses in formulating a profile of her ALDs and ALSs, and if a little alarm goes off in your head that says the goals and objectives don't fit with this picture, be sure to say so. It's always possible that these goals and objectives are being driven by existing program options or what all other students are working on in class when they must instead be based on the *individual* needs of your child.

Choosing goal areas, which set forth the desired outcome, is a lot easier than writing measurable objectives, which are defined operationally in terms of what behaviors your child will be expected to perform. This section of the IEP meeting is labor intensive. The payoff, however, for the time spent in carefully preparing the goals and objectives is that the blueprint is almost completed at this point, and you're ready to start building the foundation.

How the Goals and Objectives Are Drafted

School district staff will usually draw up a draft of goals and objectives prior to the meeting. You should do the same and/or have your consultants do so. Don't worry about this so much for your very first IEP, but after the first IEP meeting you will have a better understanding of the "goals and objectives" lingo. Ask the assessment team or the administrator in charge of scheduling the IEP meeting to let you see their draft of the goal and objectives, if available, in advance, so that your time at the meeting can be used efficiently and effectively. Ideally, the draft goals and objectives can be prepared with input from you— which might be that write-up of what you feel your child can learn in the coming year. This too will save time at the IEP meeting. By letting teachers incorporate your input before you meet formally, you may avoid some hard feelings that could come up if the team's draft hasn't included something very important to you (say, learning to eat with utensils or follow through on scheduled potty training that's working at home). In addition, Congress has also cautioned against teachers spending unnecessary time out of the classroom on irrelevant and unnecessary paperwork that does not lead to improved educational outcomes—so here's a way for you to help Congress.

Remember that as parents you are by law equal participants in the IEP process. To participate as equal members of the team, prepare as much of your own draft IEP as you can prior to the meeting. Don't worry if it isn't written in exact educational terms. At a minimum, draw up a list of goal areas important to you and a list of what you want your child to be doing in six or twelve months. For preschool children with autism spectrum disorders, especially ones who have not had much intervention before, six months may be a more reasonable measurement period.

The Importance of Being Specific

Each goal and objective must include the amount of progress required by the child—for example, 90% or 100% accuracy or correct responses on five out of five or nine of ten consecutive trials, presented across settings and with a variety of people implementing the goal and objective. Such data generally provide evidence of mastery of the goal and objective. When you first read IEPs with goals and objectives written in this manner, it may seem like some strange sort of haiku. You'll get used to it. Just try to get into the rhythm and focus of the picture it draws of your child.

Specificity in the goals and objectives is critical to the blueprint. Take a look at the following sample IEP goal and objective in one area of communication (expressive vocabulary), drafted for a preschool autistic student by the parents and their private behavioral specialist prior to the IEP meeting.

> *Goal*: To increase expressive vocabulary.
>
> *Objective*: Given a variety of group and one-on-one activities, student will increase her functional expressive vocabulary to at least 150 words, including her own name, body parts, action words, peers' names, toys, food, clothing, and animals, to be demonstrated across people and situations on a daily basis over one month, with 90% accuracy, or 4 of 5 trials, as measured by the MacArthur Communicative Development Inventory.

The first IEP goal and objective in the same area drafted by the school district team is as follows:

> *Goal*: To increase expressive vocabulary.
>
> *Objective*: Student increases her functional expressive vocabulary to 150 words.

It's easy to see the difference in specificity. In the parent/behavioral therapist goal and objective, what the student will need to learn and how and when she will need to demonstrate that knowledge are crystal clear. In the school district example, the parent and teacher will both be left with many questions about what the student needs to learn and how and when she will demonstrate that knowledge.

How Progress or Mastery Will Be Measured

You now know the baseline data, the long-term goals, the short-term objectives, and the percentage of accuracy or performance expected on each objective. But how will progress be measured?

Data collection on changes in specified behaviors and standardized tests will be the best measure of solid progress. A one-time observation is less reliable, less stable. (This goes back to the discussion we had in Part I about good-quality initial assessments using multiple sources of information to validate a potential symptom or trait.) For students who don't test well, standardized testing by an evaluator who doesn't know the child well will be problematic at best. Systematic, maybe even daily, data collection will be the most reliable measure of performance. Be sure to write in the criterion for assessing each goal and objective, if not included as a current option on the IEP form.

How Will We Get There?

Here's the meat of the matter, as far as most parents are concerned. Your child's IEP must contain a statement of the specific special education and related services and supplementary aids and services that will be provided, chosen on the basis of peer-reviewed research to the extent practicable. The services provided by the IEP have to be in effect at the beginning of each school year. If your child is between three and five years old or, at the discretion of the state educational agency, will turn three during the school year, an IFSP may serve as the IEP if consistent with state policy and agreed to by the agency and you.

Principles for Drawing the Basic Blueprint

Later in this section we'll get into the process for laying out the services provided in more detail, but first it helps to keep certain guidelines or principles in mind:

The Goal Is to Increase Your Child's Developmental Rate

Producing a substantial gain in physical development, cognitive development, language and speech, and psychosocial and self-help skills development is the goal of early intensive behavioral intervention programs, a core part of early intervention. The preschool behavioral intervention programs need to be all encompassing. Autism is, after all, just a constellation of behaviors interfering with typical development. As this book has explained, without intensive early intervention, children with autism spectrum disorders can perpetuate their own developmental delays because they may very well have no interest in learning new things simply because you want them to.

Therefore, your child may not be motivated to follow the teacher's agenda, may not be interested in learning by copying classmates, and may not be willing to stop behaving in ways that are incompatible with learning—like running around during group instruction or throwing yet-unmastered instructional materials. Each of these types of behaviors, whether direct manifestations of autistic symptoms or of failures to adapt because of autistic symptoms, must be addressed in the IEP either through curriculum adaptations and accommodations or through a behavior plan that reduces their frequency of expression so that learning can occur instead.

Programs and Placements Must Take into Account the Environment in Which Your Child Learns Most Effectively

The IDEA requires a specific written offer of program, placement, and services. The IEP cannot just state a generic "special day class" or "special education classroom" or "instructional service program." The program, placement, and services for your child must be specifically designed and determined and stated on the IEP document.

The Importance of a Home Program

Early intensive behavioral intervention programs are intended first to establish instructional control, while teaching early developmental skills that typically developing children learn from their environments without the need for specific intervention. The programs are comprehensive and focus on all of the necessary developmental skills, and they are usually delivered one to one. If the skills learned in the one-on-one setting are to be generalized across people and settings as they need to be, they should be delivered at first in the natural setting where your child is most comfortable—at home. As is discussed in Chapter 4, this is why you are essential to early behavioral intervention. On occasion, a working parent prefers to have the program and/ or services delivered at a relative's home or at day care. This certainly is appropriate if it preserves the child's access to learning skills usually learned at home—in a home, just not your child's own home. But beware of being told at your child's IEP meeting that a special day class, often an hour away by bus, *is* the only natural setting for your child. This can be a very artificial setting for your child and you; more on this below, under "Constructing the Plan." If the IEP team is truly going to plan to effect developmental change in your very young child, the home environment must be included as a place to do some significant level of work with your child. Some schools now offer intensive one-to-one teaching in a preschool special day class setting, with additional one-to-one teaching for another ten to fifteen hours per week at home. For children showing some school readiness to follow routines and generally be part of a group, this may be an appropriate middle ground.

When a Group Setting Will Be an Appropriate Environment for Learning

Clearly at some point the goal of early intervention is the generalization of skills into a group setting. The size and type of the group depends again on the individual needs of your child. Your child's program has not failed if the IEP team is considering a smaller setting than a regular education class, if that's what your child needs. You had a chance to review the advantages and disadvantages of special day classes versus general education classes as they pertain to your child's ALDs and ALSs in Chapter 7, so you know there are times when a regular education class might not be—or might be—a better environment for your child. The original goal of your early intervention plan may have been to ready your child from home for entry to a general education class. However, some children may need the extra step of a small special education class before a general education setting; other children may remain best served in special education. In any case, a careful transition must be planned, using behavioral assistants, often called "shadow aides," sometimes from your home program—if you have one—who have been trained specifically to work with your child, who know what your child can do in the one-to-one setting, and who will therefore have well-calibrated expectations that should maximally support your child's performance and interaction with peers in the new classroom. In time, your child will get to know the class, and staff will learn what your child can do and what it takes to accommodate him. At that time, the transition planning can include activities to transfer his shadowing to classroom staff. For children who still have some programming at home, however, it often makes more sense for the shadow aide to continue to be someone who can bridge both educational settings so expectations to use emerging skills are as rigorous and consistent in each setting.

How Much Is Enough Is Determined by Individual Needs

If your child is a preschooler (as well as when she's older), the parameters of appropriate programs and placements must be set based not only on the environment in which the child learns most effectively but also on how often each service should be provided and for how long a time period if it's to effect the targeted developmental changes. The law is very clear that the length of the program by day, week, month, and year must not be based on a rigid school calendar but on the individual needs of the child. The question of how much is enough has been discussed in several places earlier in this book, and Chapters 6 and 7 helped you get an idea of which needs are priorities for your child and therefore which types of treatments should take up most of the day. An individualized program plan means that you should not simply be told that "all three-year-olds get the same" ten- or twenty- (or even thirty- or forty-) hour-per-week program. If in order to obtain meaningful educational progress, your child needs a program that requires more hours than the school district typically offers to others for a special education program, such as six to eight hours a day, and even for fifty-two weeks a year, then that's what the IEP should provide. I have seen a few IEPs that even mandate services on weekends and even overnight. It can get to be a bit of a stretch to call quite this much service "educationally necessary." More important, a child with around-the-clock educationally related services is no longer being parented, and the hope that new behavior learned through these services can become part of daily living is pretty much put on hold. There are children who do need around-the-clock care that may require consistent and special skills above what parents can do. These are the types of children for whom we may consider residential care for some period to be an alternative. Most likely services will not be mandated on legal holidays (and beyond forty hours per week) unless your child *is* placed in a residential setting. Our goal is to help you obtain a program that will assist your child in becoming a productive and independent member of the community, as the federal law requires. Frequency and duration have to be based on individual needs and science-based research, not school district policy or customary practice.

Services Should Go Beyond the Traditional Therapies and Counseling

By now you know that the types of help your child needs will not be limited to traditional speech and language therapy and/or school counseling, and neither should the IEP be limited to those types of services. For example, children with autism spectrum disorders who don't develop functional verbal language skills often need visually based augmentative communication (see Chapter 8) or other tailored motivational strategies such as pivotal responding (see Chapter 7) to help them learn language and then want to use it. Remember, you're not obligated to "buy" the fixed-price menu; you can go à la carte all the way or take the multicourse meal plus some other options.

What Services Can You Request?

Behavior Intervention Specialist Services. As we've discussed, you'll want to focus on appropriate behavior intervention specialist services for designing, overseeing, and implementing an appropriate program for your child. Behavior intervention specialists are not just for solving behavior problems. Behavior specialists can be helpful in breaking down skills to be learned into necessary components, analyzing motivating strategies and reinforcers, teaching positive skills via structured peer play training, and also offering parent training so you can help your child further build these skills when he's with his family. Developing your child's prosocial behavior, play skills, and peer skills at home can and should be seen as supporting your child's ability to get the most from his classroom program. If your school does not suggest these services, but your child is of an age where things like behavior management and learning from peers are major learning issues, a case may be made that these are educationally related services. School districts may not routinely offer these services, so if you feel they might help your child get more overall benefit from his school program, you should make this a topic at your child's IEP meeting. If your child is not yet learning via direct imitation or incidental observation of peers, you'll want to discuss the need for one-on-one intervention across settings.

Extended School Year (ESY). By the fall, all children forget some of what they knew by the previous June, and in the fall teachers plan on recoupment time. For children who learn only after intensive repetition, this recoupment can be expected to take even longer. Therefore, prevention of the expected loss of skills that comes from lack of practice is more painful to watch in a child who learns more slowly. It is also a waste of precious time, especially in the first several years of life, during the period when the brain is most receptive to learning. You'll want to address the need for a twelve-month program with only reasonable breaks as appropriate to your child's rate of learning and recoupment after lack of practice. Schools generally address this concern with an extended school year program, usually offered for a four- to six-week period of summer school between June and mid-July. However, the IEP must include an individually based plan for the extended school year period for your child, not just what is available to the school district by way of general or special education classrooms and services provided in those classrooms. If you have reason to believe that recoupment is a big issue for your child, the IEP team will need to come up with alternatives to fill the gaps. This could be attendance in community-based summer programs with a shadow aide, a home-based program or more hours of a home-based program if one is already provided, or additional hours with non-school-based therapists. In the next chapter, you'll learn about what you can do during these periods to make your child's experiences meaningful and to avoid empty hours that get filled with repetitive activity.

Constructing the Plan

Now that you've established the blueprint for your child's program, you must carefully construct the levels of service and the placement that will offer the best chance of your child's making meaningful progress toward the goals and objectives in this IEP. Make sure you express concerns *now* about any behaviors of your child that tend to get in the way of learning. The IEP team has the responsibility to discuss how potential problem behaviors that interfere with learning can be handled, and you don't want to put your child (and you) through the misery of failing to "fit in" before necessary positive behavioral interventions (motivational strategies) are put in place. This might mean bringing in a behavioral specialist as part of the team, as is discussed in Chapter 8, but the IEP team has many options to make sure behavior problems don't get in the way of your child's full access to teaching resources in his program: The IEP can call for a behaviorist to simply observe your child periodically and then consult with the teacher, or, for more severe behaviors that disrupt learning, a functional behavior analysis (FBA) of a particular behavior, which will lead to a positive behavioral intervention plan.

Considering Placement Options

Your IEP team must consider a full continuum of placement options, keeping in mind that the federal law mandates that children with disabilities be taught in the least restrictive environment (LRE). At IEP meetings, you may hear team members bandying about this term LRE. What is "least restrictive" differs for each child, but it's a pivotal concept that should come up as part of your child's IEP planning. The discussion should start with the neighborhood school that your child would attend if not disabled. You need to pipe up if what is suggested as a placement does not seem to fit your child's needs or be his LRE if he is ready for a group setting. (Read the discussion in Chapter 7 about placement of your child with developmentally comparable peers so as to get the most from the curriculum.) If you're not sure what's right for your child, the team can compare the pros and cons of the proposed placement relative to placements just "above" or "below" where your child is at. A special education student is usually eligible to attend a class at schools other than his home school, so be sure you know all your choices. (The next chapter will talk about making school visits to evaluate the appropriateness of a program or classroom for your child.)

Early Intervention through Preschool

The discussion should begin with how much time services will be received in a "natural setting"—meaning either your home or a mainstream preschool. In either setting, the IEP will need to specify appropriate supports and services that will provide your child with the needed "special" part of his education. An early intensive behavioral intervention program (for example, an ABA/DTT program; see Chapter 7) is often considered a service-based special education program. This means that such a program does not *have* to be at school, nor does it always *have* to be at home. In individualizing your child's program, the IEP team, including you, needs to look at all the options. If there is no home setting where the intensive behavior intervention can be delivered, it may have to be delivered at school. Even if there is a school setting, there may be reasons related to the child's learning needs that warrant its being in the home—at least until the IEP team agrees otherwise.

As mentioned earlier in this chapter, you may encounter an opinion by a special educator that a special day class is less restrictive and, by implication, a more natural setting than home for your preschool child. But think of it this way: If your child does not learn skills sufficiently from just growing up in your home setting, as your typically developing children do, why would adding support to your home setting so that your child can develop be considered restrictive or unnatural? Is it restrictive for a blind child to use braille or a deaf child to use sign language? Must those supports be used only in special education classrooms? But blind and deaf children with otherwise typical abilities who have access to learning compensations for their disabilities while in their natural environment (their home) when they are young may never be considered candidates for special education classrooms. Our vision of creating appropriate programs, services, and supports for children with autism spectrum disorders must be broadened similarly so that as much early learning as possible can take place with the special supports of home and family.

At some point, of course, a group or school-based component *will* be necessary. One thing the classroom environment can promote is generalization of skills—applying skills learned originally in the one-on-one setting to a group setting. Another benefit of the classroom, once your child is ready for group-based learning, is that your child will be able to learn related skills spontaneously from observation of adults and peers. If all classmates are on the autism spectrum, and your child is ready to learn spontaneously and imatively, the IEP team must discuss whether your child needs this placement or a less restrictive one with peers who may be models of, and facilitators for, social interaction. This is not to contradict statements made in Chapter 7 that children don't learn how to be autistic from other autistic children. But once a child begins to demonstrate learning through spontaneous imitation, you will want her exposed to peers who are at her level or a bit higher, including typically developing peers. Special education may still be the place for more intense teaching, so you might want to look for or ask for an integrated setting with autistic and typical children, settings with socially typical but language-impaired children, or increasing amounts of time in the mainstream.

So, using the mandate for placement in the least restrictive setting as a guide, and the preceding perspective on what "least restrictive" really means for a child with autism, first the IEP team will want to discuss adding a mainstream preschool component with behavioral assistant support. This transition must be designed to succeed by gradually increasing expectations of your child and gradually fading support as appropriate. Working its way down the continuum from least to more restrictive program/placement options, the team should next consider the alternative of placing your child in a special education classroom for part or all of the instructional group-based hours. Starting with preschool special education and continuing into elementary school, the most natural and least restrictive placement might shift toward the group-based setting like this:

1. Home-based behavioral intervention program with support and services.
2. Home-based behavioral intervention program with support and services *plus* mainstream or special education classroom component with support.
3. Mainstream school or special education classroom with and/or without support *plus* home-based behavioral intervention component.

Monitoring Performance and Progress in Multiple Settings

Be aware that the transition from home-based intervention to the group-based classroom setting stands its best chance of success when information about your child's performance is shared scrupulously between you and your child's school staff. Everyone needs to be on the same page to ensure consistent and ever-increasing support for your child to do and learn new things, so at all costs you want to avoid having instructors in one setting think the child is less able than he is in another. This means someone has to keep track of what's being taught and what is being learned in each setting. While technically coordinating communication between school and out-of-school teachers and therapists is the responsibility of the school districts, in reality parents who can take on, or at least participate in, this role obtain the best outcome for their child.

As Your Child Reaches School Age

Your child's first IEP may take hours, the second one a little less. The one that moves him from preschool to kindergarten may again take more time. As your child enters the elementary grades, you'll have the same or similar discussions regarding IEPs. By elementary school, most school districts offer many fewer services at home or outside the school setting. Again, where and what services are provided depends on the individual needs of your child and must be an IEP team discussion. However, at this point, the mix of your child's year-to-year services ideally will stabilize. The rate of learning after age seven is usually more predictable from year to year. But even if the program at school is appropriate for academic learning, you need to be able to ensure that your child's social-emotional needs are met and that your child does not have empty hours where she might play video games perseveratively, watch TV shows repeatedly, or otherwise experience mental downtime as pleasurable. So the school may need to provide a homework program at school, an after-school recreation program or enrichment class(es), or adaptive sport(s) programs as part of your child's IEP. If you find yourself concerned that meaningful progress is not being achieved from the school program, you may need to advocate for more individualized instructional programs in place of or in addition to what is provided at school. But by then you should also be able to fill your child's hours with other meaningful activities, as parents do for nonautistic children.

Transitioning from School to Adulthood

At the age of sixteen, your child's IEP must include services designed to help him make the transition from school to postschool activities, including postsecondary education, vocational education, integrated employment (including supported employment), continuing and adult education, adult services, independent living, or community participation. This portion of the IEP is called the individualized transition program (ITP). As earlier in your child's educational career, these services must be based on individual needs and take into account strengths, preferences, and interests. They will still include instruction and related services to implement the IEP but also will include a vocational or functional vocational evaluation and, when needed, community-based experiences, the development of employment and other post-school adult living objectives, and/or acquisition of daily living skills.

By the time of the first IEP to be in effect after your child is sixteen, appropriate measurable postsecondary goals must be in effect based on age-appropriate transition assessments related to training, education, employment, and, where appropriate, independent living skills and the transition services (including courses of study) needed to assist the child in reaching those goals.

Assessing the IEP:
Will It Provide FAPE for Your Child?

How do you determine whether you have been offered a free and appropriate public education (FAPE)? Historically, the meaning of FAPE has been the most litigated issue since the IDEA (Individuals with Disabilities Education Act, so named in 1990) was enacted in 1975 as the Education for All Handicapped Act, the first all-encompassing federal statute governing the rights of all individuals with disabilities and the rights and obligations of school districts, county offices of education, special education local plan areas, and state departments of education.

The federal standard of appropriateness was first defined in the seminal 1982 U.S. Supreme Court case *Board of Education v. Rowley* (1982, 458 U.S. 1751) to mean "appropriate" education. In other words, the Supreme Court stated then that *appropriate* means only appropriate, and not more, unless of course you live in a state that has enacted a higher state standard and has declared a statutory intent to provide the best for each disabled child according to *Rowley*. FAPE does not mean that school districts have to maximize your child's potential unless your state requires it; it does mean, however, that school districts have to provide access to equal educational opportunities and a program that permits meaningful progress. According to cases interpreting *Rowley*, and clearly the intent of the federal statute reauthorized in 1997 and adopted in 2004 as the IDEA, school districts have to provide for your disabled student to make *meaningful* growth from year to year, while at the same time school districts have to comply carefully with the procedural protections and safeguards of what is now the IDEA.

Therefore, when trying to determine whether the IEP proposed for your child will provide him with a FAPE, you have to ask two questions:

1. Did the school district or the local educational agency (LEA) follow the procedural requirements (that is, sufficient assessment, timely and proper IEP planning) of the IDEA and, if not, was its failure so significant as to impact the educational progress of the child?
2. Is the IEP designed to allow the child to make meaningful educational progress, according to his or her potential, from year to year?

In *Rowley*, the Supreme Court held that the student did not need a sign language interpreter to achieve passing grades in general education classes. But *Rowley* was decided in the early years of implementation of the 1975 EHA. There were not a lot of children receiving early intensive behavioral intervention programs in 1982. There were not a lot of children receiving or requesting massive infusions of assistive technology services and equipment in 1982. There were not a lot of children included in the mainstream and receiving their educational programs in the so-called least restrictive environment. If we consider what's happened in the twenty-five years since the *Rowley* decision—important developments in educational programs, placements, and services available to children with disabilities; the heightened standards of IDEA 1997 and 2004; and the requirements of No Child Left Behind (NCLB)—we have to ask what it means to make progress from year to year *today*.

In addition, the standard set forth in *Rowley* has been impacted by the full inclusion movement of the 1990s. Now we have to talk about progress in a lot of different ways, not just according to test scores or passing grades but considering a whole range of factors. The evolving standard of FAPE has opened up a whole set of considerations that allows us to acknowledge that the child can be measured not only by cognitive and academic test scores, but by the ability to perform tasks outside the test situation and the ability to communicate, participate socially, and adapt to daily life situations.

Progress Must Be *Meaningful*

Significantly, even under *Rowley*, it was clear that the benefit provided in the name of facilitating the appropriate education of a child must be *meaningful*. It's very difficult to participate in an IEP meeting, or later sit in a hearing, and listen to a discussion about benefit your child has received from attending special education classes when you know that your child is not toilet trained, can't communicate his wants and needs, and runs around in the parking lot when you're trying to go to the grocery store. Meaningful benefit will be clear to you when your child progresses at least as much as relevant assessments predict. The trick here is that for progress to be meaningful, it cannot be one dimensional. Your child's program must be construed to do the best it can to plan for benefit in all areas of his development across settings. This means that teaching skills that are generalized is very important. It is not very "meaningful" if a child knows one example of each of ten animals, but when his flashcards are switched out for rubber animals, he is completely lost. Skills also need to be taught in a developmentally sensible progression: If a child still has daily toileting accidents, he should have a toileting regime on his IEP—even if he can be working on multiplication, too. It is not very meaningful if the child can read at home in a one-to-one setting but at school is only asked to work on identification of functional site words, such as "stop" and "exit."

(School staff need to be aware, too, of the importance of adherence to legally mandated procedures. Even the *Rowley* court, which set a base level standard of appropriateness, determined that where there are significant procedural violations in the development and implementation of IEPs, school districts may need to provide compensatory programs and services.)

The New Ballpark: FAPE Redefined for Preschoolers with Autism Spectrum Disorders

Most of the preschool autism spectrum disorder cases that end up in hearing have failed to adequately address the individual needs of the child and what would be meaningful progress in planning and/or implementing the IEP. There are two main reasons for this that you can address as quality assurance issues for your child's IEP: First, baseline assessments are sometimes inadequate to show where your child is starting. Second, the IEP may not include provisions for collecting enough data to know if a planned program is accomplishing what it was put in place to accomplish. You can address the former by making the contributions to the baseline discussed earlier in this chapter.

As to the second, you'll want to make sure that the IEP team thoroughly discusses how and how often your child's progress is measured. Teachers often use the term *formative evaluation* to refer to periodic testing to see how the pupil is doing and whether more or different instruction is needed. Yet if your child has received an early intensive behavioral intervention, you might be used to getting recorded data of every teaching trial the child undergoes. Understandably, special educators tell us all the time that they cannot teach with a clipboard in their hands, tallying data every second, so it's up to your child's IEP team to consider what type of data are necessary for the success of the school-based program. If a clear structure is put in place to measure progress on goals, and it is clearly understood across settings what the current functioning levels and activities are, then daily data collection may not be considered as essential as other program components, such as the training of the person doing the direct teaching.

The design of the program will be measured most appropriately by the individual response to teaching that a particular child has. That's why the courts themselves redefined FAPE for preschool autistic students in the 1990s. The research supports the fact that certain children receiving early intensive programs are better prepared for regular education classes by kindergarten or first-grade age, or at least they are able to be placed in less restrictive settings than ever contemplated for this population before the availability of early intensive intervention programs. Preschool children with disabilities consequently are now often afforded elevated rights that are similar to the goals of most early intensive behavioral intervention programs, with good reason: Obviously if you provide a very intensive program before mandatory school age, there should be a substantial saving to society. It's expensive to run special education classrooms, and even more expensive to provide custodial settings for adults who have not been educated adequately. There is an increased understanding that intensive early intervention services fulfill the goal to better prepare children on the autism spectrum for group-based learning experiences. There is additionally a moral imperative to help the youngest children to give them the greatest possible chance.

Is the IEP Supported by the Research?

The IEP process is not always structured in a way that makes parents comfortable that the school district personnel are planning for an individual program based on their individual child's needs. However, the requirement that the educational strategies and instructional programs provided for in your child's IEP be based on peer-reviewed research (see the sidebar earlier in this chapter on pages 210–211) is paramount. You have the right to insist on methods that the research has shown to be ef-

fective. To review how you can learn to distinguish peer-reviewed research from snake oil claims and everything in between, see Chapter 5.

When You Disagree with the IEP:
Legal Rights and Remedies

There are times when you simply will not agree with what the rest of
the IEP team asserts is an offer of FAPE for your child. This can happen
because of inadequate communication between parents and school
personnel. It can happen if you enter the process—or the IEP team
does—viewing the IEP planning as a kind of negotiation. From your
end, you go in with the natural position that your child is your most
valuable possession. Naturally you'll take umbrage at anyone's implication that it might not be "worth it" to give your child more of something when you believe there's a chance that it will make a critical
difference. This chapter—like the entire book—has been aimed at en-
abling you to help the IEP team understand what your child needs and
to work with the team in making that happen so that you feel you are
getting what you need.

But when you're in dispute about your request for an appropriate
research-based program for your child at the IEP level and you can't
reach agreement with your school district, you may very well have
reached the appropriate time to request a due process hearing through
the IDEA. A very difficult issue you may have to face here is, as I have
tried to explain throughout this chapter, that the law entitles you only
to an *appropriate* program for your child—one that is reasonably calcu-
lated to provide meaningful benefit—not the best possible program,
unless your state has set a higher standard. If you are considering going the due process route, get some opinions about whether the school
district has made you an appropriate offer before deciding whether to
go ahead. There are several legal tests (discussed below) that your case
must pass to prevail in a due process hearing, so consider these too.
And remember, litigation can be very stressful and time-consuming to
all involved, even if expense is not an issue.

You may have asked that your child's IEP contain *goals* that you
want but the school district refuses to include them. You can ask that
the IEP contain *services and placement* that you want but that the school
district refuses to offer or provide to your child. If you wish to reject
the school district's proposed placement and service offer and make alternative requests fo: your child, the IDEA now requires that you spe-

cifically inform the IEP team of your rejection and any intent to enroll your child in private school or private services at public expense at the child's most recent IEP meeting, or at least ten business days prior to unilaterally removing a child from public school.

Provided that you have objected to the school district's offer, and asked for alternative programming at an IEP meeting before removing your child from school, or provided notice in writing at least ten business days ahead of removing your child, you can also ask for *reimbursement for private placements and services* that you have provided for your child with a disability because of the disputed IEP. However, reimbursement is available only for programs you have provided for your child in the absence of appropriate offers from the school district. If you have been unable, or only partly able, to provide outside programs or services, you can also ask for compensatory education or services to make up for lost educational opportunity or benefit. If you don't inform the IEP team, or at least provide ten business days' written notice to the district of this intent, a court or hearing officer may later limit or deny your reimbursement for such private school or private service expenses.

A court or hearing officer may also now limit or deny retroactive reimbursement for the unilateral placement of your child in private school or private services if prior to the removal of your child the district informed you of its intent to evaluate the child and you didn't make your child available for assessment, or if, for any reason, the court or hearing officer makes a finding that you've acted unreasonably.

However, a court or hearing officer may *not* limit or deny reimbursement to parents if the school district prevented you from providing such notice, or you didn't receive prior written notice from the school district of their refusal to provide what you requested (see below), or if compliance with the notice provisions would likely result in physical harm to your child. At the discretion of the court or a hearing officer, reimbursement may not be reduced or denied for failure to provide such notice if you were illiterate or couldn't write in English or compliance would result in serious emotional harm to your child.

The school district is required to provide you with Prior Written Notice (a formal document) whenever it proposes to initiate or change, or refuses to initiate or change the identification, evaluation, or educational placement of your child, or the provision of a free appropriate public education to your child. These laws are designed in the spirit of how the IEP process should work—which is everyone keeping everyone else apprised of what they are thinking and the reasoning behind it. If you do become involved in a filing for due process, you need to know that the Prior Written Notice must include:

- A description of the action proposed or refused by the agency;
- An explanation of why the agency proposes or refuses to take the action and a description of each evaluation procedure, assessment, record, or report the agency used as a basis for the proposed or refused action;
- A statement that as the parents of a child with a disability you are protected under the procedural safeguards section . . . and, if this notice is not an initial referral for evaluation, the means by which you can obtain a copy of a description of the procedural safeguards;
- Sources for you to contact to obtain assistance in understanding the provisions;
- A description of other options considered by the IEP team and the reason those options were rejected; and
- A description of the factors that are relevant to the agency's proposal or refusal.

If your state does not have its own statute on the time frame for filing an action when you have a dispute, the IDEA of 2004 sets forth a two-year statute of limitation on raising your claims from the date you or the agency knew or should have known of the action forming the basis of the complaint. However, the timeline does not apply to you if you were prevented from requesting the hearing due to (1) specific misrepresentations by the local educational agency (LEA) that it had resolved the problem forming the basis of the complaint or (2) the LEA's withholding of information from the parent that was required under the notice provision. Since each state may have its own statute of limitations on reimbursement, you should ask about the length of time prescribed by the statute in your own state.

A little-used remedy by parents or parent representatives is to seek direct services by the state educational agency if the local educational agency or school district is unable to establish or maintain FAPE. For example, if your school district refuses to offer or provide an early intensive intervention program, give notice to your state department of education (DOE) of your request for the programming and of your intent to seek reimbursement from the state DOE for the costs of the program if you can start it yourself.

Do You Need Legal Assistance?

This is a complicated process. Where can you find skilled advocacy assistance or an attorney? Each state has a federally mandated and funded advocacy center to represent the developmentally disabled. Even where they are not able to provide individual services to clients, they are excellent resources and often have extensive referral lists and in-service programs for IEP preparation. Parent network groups, such as FEAT, are great resources for service referral as well and potentially great support for new families after receiving the diagnosis of ASD.

Can you seek reimbursement for the fees and costs of a lawyer to represent your child? Since 1986, attorneys for students have been entitled to payment by school districts for reasonable attorney's fees when parents obtain a favorable outcome for their children in IDEA disputes. However, the United States Supreme Court has recently ruled that this reimbursement for attorney's fees does not include expert fees or costs. A further caveat is that if the school district makes a formal written offer to settle the case at least ten days prior to the hearing, and you don't obtain a decision that provides you with a remedy worth more than the offer, you won't be entitled to reimbursement for your attorney's fees and costs.

If you lose your due process case, do you have to pay the school district attorney's fees and costs? In 2004, Congress added a provision for the first time that state educational agencies or local school districts considered prevailing parties may be awarded reasonable attorney's fees if the administrative complaint or court action is or becomes frivolous, unreasonable, or without foundation, or was presented for any improper purpose, such as to harass, to cause unnecessary delay, or to needlessly increase the cost of litigation.

Can you file a case in court if you have a dispute? Yes, but first you have to exhaust administrative remedies. This means you have to go through the due process or administrative hearing first and then appeal if you feel the administrative judge or hearing officer has made a mistake. Keep in mind that this chapter does not focus on children who qualify only for Section 504 of the 1973 Rehabilitation Act or the 1990 Americans with Disabilities Act. There may also be remedies available under Section 504 for your child, as all students who qualify for an IEP also qualify for Section 504 protections; however, you must also exhaust administrative remedies to bring a Section 504 claim. Examples of Section 504 claims that would ordinarily not be brought under IDEA cases would be claims related to damages for teacher or student harassment, claims related to providing equal access to neighborhood schools when physical barriers prevent school attendance, or claims for damages for discrimination based on disability. Teacher or student harassment, access, and discrimination issues may also be reasons why FAPE is not provided to your child under your IDEA case.

What Happens When You Request a Due Process Hearing?

The school district must reply within ten days to a parental complaint or request for a hearing. Notwithstanding this reply, within fifteen days, the school district must inform the hearing office if it is asserting that the parental hearing request is not "sufficient." In the event that this occurs, the judge or hearing officer must review the complaint and determine whether it is sufficient or insufficient to proceed to a hearing within five days of receipt of the notice of insufficiency.

Also within fifteen days of the filing of the complaint or request for hearing, the school district must hold a resolution session to discuss and attempt to resolve your dispute. While the school district can decide to waive this session, you cannot waive it by yourself without agreement from the school district. Since the district is required to have only IEP team members present at the resolution session, including personnel with authority to resolve the issues, if you have already had protracted IEP-level meetings without a successful agreement for your child's program, placement, and services, you may want to ask that the session be waived by agreement and that a mediation be scheduled instead.

At a mediation, a skilled mediator can assist the parties with resolution. An additional reason to consider agreeing to a waiver of the resolution session and requesting mediation instead, especially if an attorney is representing you, is that no attorney's fees can be awarded for representation at the resolution session. One caveat to remember is that both parties must be willing to participate in a mediation, as it is voluntary, and not mandatory under the IDEA. However, if a mediation process is agreed to, a mediated agreement can be the most effective and expedient way to govern the outcome for your child's educational program, as you, and not an outside judge or hearing officer, will have control over the outcome.

If your case does not settle, five business days before the hearing, that is, seven days in advance of the hearing, you must provide to the school district and the hearing office formal disclosures of your hearing issues and proposed resolutions; formal notice of the documents you wish to present as evidence at the hearing, including copies of the documents; and a formal notice of or list of the witnesses you wish to call on your behalf to testify at the hearing and the subject or areas of their testimony, including expert witnesses.

Can the School District Itself Request a Hearing?

Yes, and the party it requests the hearing against will be your child. This can be a very intimidating event. You may feel that you cannot adequately represent yourself in such a circumstance. Please refer to the Resource section at the end of this book for referrals for help in representing your child if this occurs. The same timelines pertain to you should the school district file for hearing: You must respond within ten days to the complaint or request for hearing and must let the hearing office know if you believe that the complaint or request for hearing is insufficient within fifteen days. One important difference is that no resolution session is required when it's the school district that files for hearing. Mediation is still available, but again both parties must be willing to participate in the mediation since it's voluntary and not mandatory.

What Happens When There's a Due Process Hearing?

These due process hearings generally are held at the local school district office or a local public building where you reside. You can request that the hearing be held in a public building other than your district office if that location is intimidating to you or inconvenient to your witnesses. Prior to hearing, mediation must be available, if the parties agree to participate, even if it's before parties request due process. Mediation must be voluntary and cannot be used to deny a parent's right to due process or to deny any other rights under federal law and must be conducted by an impartial mediator trained in effective mediation techniques. An experienced mediator can assist you and the school district in facilitating an agreement to resolve the disputes. In California, according to the statistics released by the Special Education Hearing Office prior to July 1, 2005, approximately 95% of the cases filed actually settled in mediation, which is encouraging. A case that doesn't settle in mediation then proceeds to the due process hearing at the local school district.

What If You Don't Win Your Case?

Either side can appeal the hearing decision to court. Generally, a case is appealed to federal court, because the IDEA is a federal statute. The parties don't have the right to a full trial de novo (an all-new trial) on appeal, but do have the right to supplement the evidence, according to the statute, and the court must conduct a substantial review of the record and make a decision based on a preponderance of the evidence. Under the IDEA, damages are generally limited to reimbursement for placement, services, and programs already provided unilaterally by parents or requests for compensatory services or programs. However, the statute permits any remedy the court deems appropriate. Please note that in some states the hearing process is a two-tiered system, and you must in that case appeal to the state review officer before appealing to court. You must review your parental rights statements and/or contact your local or state school agencies or local advocacy agencies or consultants to see which hearing system your state has chosen to provide and how to proceed.

Who Has the Burden of Proof at the Hearing?

The United States Supreme Court, the highest court in the land, has determined that it is the party seeking to change the IEP who has the burden of proof at the hearing. This means that if you are seeking to change your child's IEP, you may have the burden of proving that the school district offer, or implemented program, does not provide your child with FAPE and that your requested placement and services should be provided to implement the IEP instead, or that you should receive the reimbursement requested for what you have provided yourself, or that your child should receive the compensatory education requested from the school district. This also means that your school district may have the burden of proving that its request to change your child's IEP, placement, and/or services will provide an FAPE to your child.

When I began to practice law in this field, I saw many autistic students placed in institutions by adolescence, if not before, no matter what their potential was or what type of private or public special class placement had been provided. The problem was that the interventions were not intensive enough, were not provided early enough, and were not specifically designed to significantly change the developmental rate to foster reaching full potential. It has only been since the 1990s

What If You Move?

If your child transfers school districts and enrolls in a new school within the same state in the middle of the school year, your new school district must provide services comparable to those described in the previous active IEP to ensure that he still gets an FAPE. The district must consult with you and must continue providing these services until it either adopts the previous IEP or develops a new one consistent with federal and state law. If your child is transferring from a different state, the local educational agency (LEA) must provide the comparable services in consultation with you until the LEA conducts an evaluation, if the agency considers one necessary, and develops a new IEP if appropriate.

that the meaning of providing free and appropriate public education (FAPE) to the autistic preschool population has been redefined to include the provision of early intensive intervention programs, and families all over the country have clamored to obtain programming for their children with autism spectrum disorders, thus impacting the future development of an entire population. Congress has agreed with the need for high expectations and effective research-based methodologies to assist your child to reach academic achievement and functional performance so that he or she can lead an independent and productive life. Educators as well as parents and treating professionals should be proud of the results their collaborative efforts are creating.

TEN

Sharing the Driving

THE RIGHTS AND RESPONSIBILITIES
OF A COLLABORATIVE PARENT

In the last chapter, you learned all about your child's legal rights to education from someone who has championed those rights for children with autism. In most areas of civil rights, though, we don't just speak of rights—we speak of rights and responsibilities. This means that the benefits that society confers come with a responsibility to act within certain limits and engage in negotiation to arrive at mutual understandings that give rise to mutual benefit. What I'm talking about is a two-way street. How do you work most successfully with providers in a mutually respectful and mutually beneficial way? How do you do this without maximizing your own stress levels?

Right now, in the field of special education, relations between parents and schools are not always ideal. The litigation that has brought rights has too often also brought a sense of absolute right and wrong. Usually it's the parent who feels wronged, has brought suit, and then has had that view upheld by a legal decision. That probably doesn't mean everything the school did was wrong, however. It also doesn't mean that everything the wronged parents want now is right or righteous. Very often, though, this sense of "I was right, and you were wrong, and now you'll pay" seems to become the ethos of subsequent interactions between parents and those with the educational purse strings. But these educators are also those most centrally positioned to help. You may have a nonpublic program today—or tomorrow—but your child is going to need an education until he's grown. Whether your child is in private special education paid for with public funds or public special or general education, you are going to have to deal with "the system." Thinking "I'll bring my lawyer along!" is no way to set out if we are all to act in the *best interest of the child*. It is also no way to act if you are to maintain your equilibrium, your marriage (if you're in one), and the mental health of the rest of your family.

From where I am—and, I hope, anyone else reading this is—coming from, acting in the best interest of the child is the name of the game. It's the *only* game. In this chapter, we will all learn to play nicely. This means that even when you're feeling hurt and are anxious for and about your child, you'll treat everyone else involved with your child like they have feelings too—because they do. This means that educators and therapists will not behave paternalistically, as if they know it all—because they don't. It means that "experts" and folks like me who try to call the shots must admit we're not dealing with a "my way or the highway" situation. Any plan for treatment, any treatment decision, needs to be formed jointly by the professional who knows all sorts of things about treatment and you, the parent, who knows all sorts of things about "reading" and motivating your particular child. Collaboration is essential to the success of any child's treatment.

As I've already said in a number of ways in earlier chapters, there is no *one* right way. We need solutions that work for everyone, with the child—no one else—at the head of the queue. So let's explore some ideas for getting along in a manner that is sustaining—and not crazy-making.

Today Is the First Day of the Rest of Your Life . . .

Now you've learned all about the IEP process. You know your rights. You know that your child is entitled to a free and appropriate public education. The things parents find themselves thinking about as they move into the implementation of their child's first IEP can be quite varied. Emotions can be expected to shift rapidly. Whenever people face new, complex, and unfamiliar life events, emotions are unsettled.

When your child starts out as an "official" part of a new world of help and helpers, part of you can feel like your baby is being taken away from you. There is no human drive stronger than the desire to protect one's baby.

Some parents are completely trusting: These parents are positively impressed by the people who offer ways to help their child. I would like to think that most people warrant the trust they command. But some parents are understandably more suspicious. They have been sensitized by long, drawn-out negotiations prior to the start of any treatment. They may have had the experience of already-withdrawn promises. Be aware of where you are on this continuum with respect to each of the people who will be helping your child.

Don't prejudge. First impressions don't always tell the tale. Be open, try to trust—but expect trust to be earned if it's to be retained.

Some parents are naturally more secure than others. Security is partly personality but definitely influenced by having the money to make choices, having the education to understand the pros and cons of choices, feeling that the educators are part of the same community as you, and many other factors. Keep your personal like or dislike for someone separate from rational decision making. Keep any natural bias that something must be better for your child if it costs more separate from rational decision making. Keep any fear that you may be getting less than the best for your child if you rely 100% on publicly funded services separate from rational decision making.

When it's time to implement a child's first IEP, some parents proceed full-speed ahead; others want to run and hide. Neither extreme is likely to be best for your child: The parent who wants to push an ABA/DTT program up to thirty hours a week as quickly as possible needs to take a look at how the child is handling things and let that govern the pace. Conversely, if you think your child "just isn't ready"—to leave you, go to school, spend time with new people, have limits set, whatever—you too may risk confusing those feelings of your own with your child's reactions. Try to separate yourself from your child and move ahead based on the child's responses.

Some parents start out optimistic that things can only get better. Usually this is the case. But getting better does not always look better from that first moment. A child who begins a new treatment can experience it as things going topsy-turvy. A new world order. Not necessarily bad, but new. New things take time for accommodation and adjustment. Recognize that your child very well may be unhappy when the status quo gets changed. Hang in there. Don't get pessimistic because your first week of therapy does not produce your child's first word or first sentence. Don't let your disappointment that things aren't going faster leave you with a perpetually half-empty cup. Listen (and try to feel joy!) when someone tries to point out the new things your child has begun to do and understand.

Playing Nicely = Mutual Respect

The roller coaster of parental emotions—from trusting to suspicious, secure to insecure, eager to hanging back, optimistic to pessimistic—may seem like just what you don't need right now. It's going to happen, though. Know that it's normal. Try to separate what's happening to your feelings from what is happening to your child. Years after a first diagnosis of autism, many parents can talk about how this was a sad, anxious, even angry period of their lives when fear of the future, self-blame, and just being overwhelmed made it near impossible to be the good person they wanted to be for the loved ones in their lives.

When your apprehensions spill out, there are a few places they can go where they probably won't do any good: They can spill all over your child. If you show your anxiety, he's going to be more anxious too. If you come into a classroom or therapy room and clutch your child more tightly, he'll feel it—and react. Your apprehensions can rub off on your child's teacher, tutor, or therapist. This too may be counterproductive; helping your child has got to come from a collaborative process with these folks, and collaboration starts with being able to put yourself in their shoes. Almost all the helping professionals will want to do the best job for your child that they can. They really will need *your* help to get to know your child—so they can begin to apply what they know.

When you're so worried about finding the right person to entrust your child to, how do you muster the forbearance it might take as a new provider gets to know your child and gets into the groove of teaching him? First of all, realize that no one goes into special education to get rich—or famous. For the privilege of having spent four years in college, completing teacher credentialing courses, interning for six months for free, and often completing a master's degree, a special education teacher can earn a salary similar to a department manager at Macy's. So why do special educators do what they do for a living? They do it because, by and large, each therapist or educator hopes to make a difference in the quality of a child's life—and, if you're lucky, in the quality of the child's family's life. (Does this help to explain why teachers can be so sensitive when told that they know *nothing* if they haven't flown to Texas and been to the same $3,500 RDI weekend workshop that you have?)

But what if your child has been having daily child-led play sessions at home based on the RDI approach, and it has helped her language and nonverbal communication? You definitely want to continue it, but it seems the school staff is not prepared to use that model. Do you (1) file a lawsuit for "stay put" in your home program, (2) insist that the RDI therapist, who is not a credentialed teacher, come to class and "train" the teacher, (3) just hope and trust that whatever the school does is going to be okay, even though you don't see how, or (4) figure out how to discuss and negotiate a compromise position everyone can live with?

Teachers in particular are in a difficult position when it comes to juxtaposing the needs of the child, the child's parents, who act on their child's behalf, and the school administration—who must act on behalf of all children equally. You're responsible only for making sure your child gets what she needs. The school administration is mandated to serve all children equally well and, of course, not to engage in any kind of favoritism. The teacher is somewhere in between, identified with both the parents' and school's positions. The teacher feels responsible and righteously proud of each new thing she can help a child in her class achieve—just like a parent does. The teacher also feels responsible for ensuring that *every* child in her class gets what he as an individual needs and that no child gets more at another's expense.

On top of this, teachers can be under pressure to fall in line with a school philosophy (like full inclusion) or budgetary mandates (like no more than one-to-three staffing). If the teacher is seen as bucking the system, she may be compromising her own status and job security in the teaching hierarchy. For example, your child's teacher may realize that he could access instruction much more of the time or lose less time to disruptive behavior if he had a one-to-one aide. A school administrator might in fact see where this is true—but also be aware of several other children in other classes who could similarly benefit from more individualized instruction. If the administrator gives in to your child's teacher's request for an additional aide, other teachers may see it as an opportunity to ask as well or may see your child's teacher as being favored (or themselves as disfavored).

What do *you* do? If you have a good relationship with your child's teacher, you can begin to talk about it. Is there a way of deploying aide time better? Could a parent volunteer do some of the managerial things that an aide does (like taking kids to therapy, the bathroom, or setting up for snack)? Could your child get more one-to-two time with a staff member if not one-to-one? Could he be paired with a very similar student who needs to be learning the same things in a similar way? If there was one more aide for the class, how could that person's time help everyone? Does the teacher think it would help if two or three parents got together and asked the administrator for something that would benefit more than one child?

The point is that if you want a problem addressed, you need to show a willingness to contribute to the solution. And that means starting with a set of positive assumptions about your child's teacher (or therapist) and building up expectations for that individual from there. If you assume your child's helping professional is less than competent, that person will have no motivation to do his best for you or your child. (This is the "you will catch more flies with honey than vinegar" principle.) Before the school year or therapy arrangement starts, meet with this person. Ask about his training and experience. Ask what he knows or has heard or done with different kinds of therapeutic approaches you feel may help your child. Listen to what he has to say and learn what his ideas are founded on. Learn what kinds of experiences the professional has had and then think about which ones might help him help your child. What made him get into teaching children with autism? Does he have a family member who's autistic? Does he have kids of his own? Is he married? Where does he live? Learn about him. Then tell him something about who you are and who your child is.

Put yourself in the position of a first-year teacher. You are given a big empty room, a few desks and tables, a couple of movable walls, some closets, and, if you are lucky, a computer or two. Maybe you inherit some old toys and books from a retiring teacher or the last occupant of this classroom. You are given about five hundred dollars to buy supplies for the year. How do you make this into a place where children can learn? How do you make this into a place you will be eager to come to each day? How do you make this into a place where parents can look around and have confidence that you know what you are doing?

Teachers and therapists need to put a tremendous amount of thought and time into creating an environment for learning. Your child's teacher or therapist is someone for whom you must show respect from the get-go. In this country, you are innocent till proven guilty. Perhaps saying such a thing about a teacher would have been unnecessary twenty-five years ago. Today it is not. This is the crux of the "rights and responsibilities" issue. Yes, you as a parent of a child with special needs have rights, but it is your responsibility to do everything you can to support the efforts of the teachers and others trying to afford your child the best treatment possible.

There will be times you may end up with a teacher or therapist who is not up to snuff. Teachers leave job commitments at the last minute, get married and move, or go on maternity leave. A new teacher may need to be found fast, and may not be as good as one that could have been found through a longer hiring process. You might end up with a speech and language therapist or other therapist covered by your insurance who doesn't know her way around autism—and even says so up front. If you need to change your services away from this provider, make a list of specific concerns before you take it to the next level: For example: "Visual augmentative communication has been recommended for my child, and this speech and language therapist uses only sign language for preverbal children." Or "This teacher teaches only in groups so the children can learn by imitating each other, and my child doesn't imitate; I've been told that's why he needs lots of one-to-one direct, behaviorally based teaching right now." Statements such as these proactively state what you're looking for, not just what you don't like. They give the administrator a sense of where you want to go. Also, remember how in Chapter 8 we talked about how a child's motivation is improved by giving him choices? Well, the school administrator's motivation might just also be improved by giving *him* choices of where you see things as being able to go from here.

Making Observations in Classrooms

To know what your child will get, or what your child is getting, you may need to plan one or more classroom visits. What will you look for to know whether a class is offering needed learning resources for your child? When you step into a new classroom, think about all that went into creating it. Think about the teacher who made it happen. Little fairies didn't come in at night and get it organized. The classroom is the window into a teacher's soul as an educator. To be in her class is to experience something quite personal about her.

A great deal goes into organizing a classroom to make it a place where children can learn. It's important for you to know what to look for so that you have some idea about the fit between a classroom or therapist and your child. One dimension of analyzing a classroom is to recognize the approaches being used. Another dimension is to understand whether what you're seeing (say a DTT program, a TEACCH class, or Floortime) indeed is what it is said to be. A third dimension involves the resources for implementation: Through conversations with the involved professionals, you'll need to weigh whether they can deliver what they promise. An excellent teacher who has too many children or not enough staff, or a fine therapist who really doesn't have time in her schedule, may not work out as well as someone who lacks the same track record but is very interested in learning as she goes. Good therapy or good teaching is partly an art that involves getting to know your subject. Until a helping professional begins to work with a child, it may be hard to know with complete certainty what the fit will be.

Going to See Classes or Therapists with a "Docent"

I don't know about you, but when I go to a museum or gallery to see postmodern art of any sort, it helps me to have an audio guide, a docent, or a knowledgeable friend along. Without guidance, I often don't have a clue what I am looking at, what else a piece may be informed by, or what in the world the artist may have been thinking, feeling, or trying to say by creating the piece. Sad to say, I think it is a pretty normal human reaction to dislike that which is incomprehensible—which, when I am unaided, is often how I end up reacting to postmodern art. For many parents, visiting your first special education classroom, observing an ABA/DTT program, or seeing a speech therapist use pictures to teach communication can elicit a similar set of responses: "I don't know what this is; I can't tell if it's any good; it doesn't grab me intuitively; I dislike it." So, it can be helpful to have help when you try to do this.

What you may want to consider is seeing classrooms with a pro. Logically, you would want to visit programs or therapists with someone who knows a program but doesn't have a vested interest in it. For example, having another mother invite you over to see how great her ABA program is is fine—for her. Your child may be at a different point developmentally, learn differently, or have different chemistry with these tutors. The same is true of an ABA agency showing you a program of one of its high responders. Not that you shouldn't avail yourself of these opportunities; you should—but with an open mind. Similarly, going to see a classroom with a school district staff person can have limitations. You may be steered to a specific class because it really is the best fit or for more extraneous reasons such as that other classes are "filled" (that is, would require hiring additional teachers or aides), require more complex busing arrangements, and so forth. Conversely, some school district personnel will show parents many classes and therapists, some of which are unbelievably irrelevant—just to make the point that you are being given choices. Lovely. Don't waste your time on that.

For a successful program visit, consider taking along a clinician from a diagnostic or assessment clinic who is familiar with the treatment models you will consider. Let's assume that anyone who has recommended, say, a DTT program for your child knows what a good DTT program looks like when she sees one. In many locales, there are educational consultants who offer the service of evaluating programs for parents. Such specialists are invaluable in finding the right match between your child and those with the best skill set to address your child's individual needs. Don't bother to hire anyone who doesn't want you to come along. Also don't hire a specialist who has likely already decided that any program (other than the one he offers) will be inadequate. Let's face it. If you pretty much know what such an evaluator will say about a school program, it's a waste of your money and time to go see the program with that person. You want someone who understands that her job as a program evaluator is to identify the services that will be the best fit for your child. Even if the class or service is not right, you should learn something from learning why not, or what a good version of the service for your child would look like— aside from the service this evaluator might herself provide.

Why Observation Visits Are Important

Getting to know a service, therapy, or program before agreeing to enroll your child is important for several reasons. First, of course, you want to see what the program or therapy is about and, importantly, if it is likely to be a good fit for your child. Second, you want to develop an understanding of how you as a parent can interface with what this school, program, or therapist would be doing with your child. Third, by just showing up to make an observation, you present yourself as someone who desires to be proactive in your child's development.

In many ways making a visit to a program or therapist is a way of introducing yourself before you make the decision about whether you want to introduce your child. Should you take your child along? I almost always think this is a less than wonderful idea for a first visit to a group-based program. Why? It's confusing to your child to meet people just once who may either turn out to be very important or whom he'll never see again. Also, a child's reaction to a new person and/or new place is no basis for judging whether you've found a good place for your child to learn. Autistic children have too many problems with things that are new and out of the routine, let alone adults who are new and exposure to social settings with peers who are new.

By going alone to a first contact visit, you emphasize that the adult-to-adult relationship is important to you. What's your impression of this therapist or teacher as a person? Does she seem like a person with whom you'd be comfortable chatting? Is she someone with whom you can have a respectful conversation where you both lay out ideas, listen to each other, and respond?

Sometimes visiting a program is impractical because it interferes excessively with another child's treatment. This can be the case if you are looking to choose a speech and language therapist or a provider for an in-home ABA/DTT program. In this case, an alternative is to view a program remotely. You can do this by viewing videotapes or DVDs of a therapy session or classroom or by observing via a video camera with remote monitor or through a one-way mirror. If you're going to watch a video of another child's therapy, the teacher or therapist is, of course, going to have to get the consent of that child's parent first. It should be a child with learning needs similar to your child's. If you observe through a mirror or monitor, you will need your docent and/or the therapist/teacher there to discuss what you're seeing. If you can watch a program along with the teacher or the therapist while other staff work with children, you'll test the waters about what it might be like to have this professional working with your child.

What to Ask Yourself (or Your Docent) during an Observation

When you reach the point where you are going to make decisions about whom to involve in your child's treatment, you may just feel desperate to get started. Early in this book we discussed how earlier *is* better but also that earlier may *not* be better if what you are doing is not really what your child needs most. This means that you need to get the right services but get them expeditiously. The best way to proceed is to start off with some criteria in mind. Some of these criteria may help you decide whether a class or therapist is even worth investigating in person. Other criteria prepare you for what you need to look for when you make a visit.

Here are some criteria for selecting classes or therapists to visit in choosing a program or therapist for your child.

Are the other children within a couple years of your child's chronological age? Children under three are usually in their own programs; three- to five-year-olds are grouped together; early elementary (six- to eight-year-olds) are together; older elementary (nine- to eleven-year olds) are together; and middle-schoolers and high-schoolers are together. If your child is exceptionally small or exceptionally large physically, there is no reason he has to be with chronological agemates. "Grade" as far as special education classes go is a pretty fluid concept, so don't let that steer you away from a teacher who you feel can still or might otherwise benefit your child.

Are the other children within a couple of years of your child developmentally? If your child is not talking yet, you need to think twice about what your child can access from a class where most or all the others are talking in phrases or sentences. Conversely, if your child is easily speaking in long utterances (even if echolalic), she may not be a good fit in a classroom filled with visual supports for every child. While visual supports can help verbal children get organized, a verbal child is not going to need a class where pictures are the expressive coin of the realm.

Is this class equipped to handle highly disruptive behavior? This is a two-part question: First, are there disruptive pupils in the class? Are any outbursts handled in a way that circumvent disruption of the instruction of others? If so, fine. Second, if you have a child with behaviors that interfere with his instruction, you will want to see examples of similar behavior being handled in a manner that does not compromise instruction time—for him or for others. Unfortunately, one bad apple can spoil the barrel. A teacher who does not have skills, a behavior plan, or appropriate staffing to handle disruptive behavior can end up with a class that is disadvantageous to most of the pupils in it.

Does this classroom or therapist offer the methods you have been told it does? Do the methods seem implemented with fidelity? Is the content of the program, given the method, appropriate for the child's developmental level? For example, if you are seeing a TEACCH program for a child who can read sentences and point to main objects described in a caption, his workstation tasks might include matching captions to pictures (not just matching objects to like objects). This is to say that it's important to observe not just whether the methods are used correctly but also whether they are well geared to where each child is at. Of course, you won't have explicit information about other children in a class but should have a sense of whether a child is bored by things being too simple or frustrated by things being over his head. You should also have a sense of whether the therapist or teacher can see where a child is—and adjust accordingly. You can get this information from your own observations, from those of your docent or expert, and from talking to the teacher or therapist about what she was thinking as she worked with a particular child.

Do you like being in this place? A classroom I visited some years ago had a needlepointed plaque above the door that read "Welcome to Where My World Makes Sense." When you visit a class or observe a therapist in action, that's the epitome of what you are looking for. A great teacher or therapist is one who becomes the child's "interpreter" while pulling back just enough to encourage the child's own "fluency." A class where a teacher is really great at this can feel like a mini–United Nations, with each child speaking a different language or dialect but the teacher changing how she addresses each child according to his needs. Most parents can feel this instinctively. However, if you'd like some rational criteria too, here are some: As you walk around a classroom, is there an indication that some materials are specific for each child? Are they sufficiently visual versus language based? Is instructional content built around what motivates the child? Are the materials something fun to handle that would make a child like yours eager to get to them? Does each child have some things or places that are her own? For example, an individual speech and language pathologist might have a little basket with specific materials for each child she sees. A special day classroom might have a particular area for each child. An inclusion setting may have a place for the child that is thoughtfully located near the teacher and natural peer helpers, as well as apart from natural peer victimizers and sources of potential distraction—like a shared computer station.

In the case of children with autism, the classroom must have developmentally appropriate accessible materials, but not enough access to be overstimulating. Things that are rewarding to the child, such as toys with strong sensory properties, can be excellent teaching materials—in moderation. Most special day classes have areas defined for whole group, small group, and individual work activities. If you're looking at some form of inclusion and plan to do it with a shadow aide, you should learn about how and where the aide will spend time in the classroom so that she physically does not overshadow the child—but also is integrated as a classroom helper at times and in ways that enable her to be seen as an asset to the teacher and active in other classroom activities if your child is doing just fine on his own. (This latter is important because it allows the shadow to be seen as something other than your child's personal handmaiden—which tends to exclude rather than include your child in the activities of his peers.)

Dos and Don'ts of Classroom Observation Etiquette

There definitely are ground rules to be followed in any visit to a potential program or therapist: First, you should inquire what the rules for visiting are—and how you might subscribe to them. This shows your "earnest money" with respect to being a collaborator with those who will help your child learn. I've known a few parents who expect schools to welcome or even tolerate snap "inspections." Public schools are not the military, and you certainly are not the camp commandant. Yes, you are the taxpayer, but so are the teachers, the principal, and the parents of all the other students. A good policy is for schools to have assigned times of day for visits when a school staffer such as a resource teacher, autism content specialist, or speech therapist is available to accompany you. These visits usually commence after all the pupils have arrived and a designated activity is scheduled.

It's also a good idea to meet the teacher and see the physical environment of the classroom when class is not in session. The best way to do this is before you actually observe in a class. This might be for fifteen to thirty minutes before class starts or on a day prior to a classroom or therapy visit. Before pupils arrive (or after they leave) is the best time to see the materials in a classroom. Teachers are usually happy to give guided tours of their domain. This is a good time to ask questions about methods used in the class, but be prepared to hear not just yes or no, but a rationale for "how," "with whom," "when," and "where." A good example of this is a parent who might ask, "Do you do discrete trials?" The teacher might say, "No, but we do intensive one-to-one teaching that is individualized to each child's IEP requirements." If you are looking for a class that does offer one-to-one teaching, and what you should look for has been characterized to you as "discrete trials," you will need to look carefully before you rule such a class in or out. Teachers who have been trained in pivotal response or incidental teaching (discussed in Chapter 7) may say no to DTT because they rightfully consider what they do to be more modern technologically. You should be more interested in whether the teacher can walk the walk than in whether she can talk the talk.

As the first bus arrives at 8:00 A.M., be prepared to say a quick thank-you and good-bye unless you have arranged to stay on and observe. If the first bus comes at 7:55, you'll be leaving early—because when the kids arrive, the teacher needs to get to work. If you haven't finished asking your questions, you can always arrange to call a teacher after school to learn more about what you saw in an observation—or ask whoever else from the school might also be along on your visit. Keeping to prearranged guidelines shows respect for a teacher's work. Even if you don't like the teacher or class, the respect is "money in the bank" for further negotiations.

Most schools require that someone from the school accompany you on observations. This requirement is not intended, as I have sometimes heard it construed, mainly to make sure you don't see anything untoward. It's meant to ensure that you understand the practices in place. It's fine, in fact very helpful, to have your docent along for any meetings with school staff as well as an actual classroom visit. You can meet with him after the visit concludes to better understand what sense he made of what the two of you were told by school staff, observed of the teacher, and observed of a classroom. The same format can be used if you are going to see an ABA/DTT program. If you are going to see a speech and language pathologist or an occupational therapist, there may be a practice partner or intern who can show you around or talk with you while you observe a session together.

Developing Proactive Relationships with Those Who Help Your Child

Effective strategies for building good working relationships between your family and your child's therapists and teachers are well worth learning and implementing as you pick specific providers of help for your child and negotiate your child's IEP. Once you've selected services and service providers, your family is ready to embark on this special education adventure. We'll discuss some things to consider to keep things working smoothly.

An Apple for the Teacher?

When your child starts to learn, it may seem fairly apparent which professionals are most strongly associated with the child's successes. This naturally buoys your respect and admiration for this person. Parents who see their child learning readily for the first time want to give their thanks. How best to show your appreciation? How do you make your thanks into a gift that keeps on giving?

The first issue is recognizing the source of a child's benefit. Too often, parents who have a child in a home program and at school say to me, "I know the home program is where he learns. I'm only sending him to school for 'socialization.'" To play the devil's advocate here, I find myself wondering if that's because this parent sees the home program on a daily basis but rarely sees much of the school program. There is nothing more wondrous than observing a "eureka" moment when your child forges ahead and solves a problem he couldn't even begin to attack earlier. Not surprisingly, the therapist or teacher who guides your child through that moment is seen as some sort of miracle worker. Could there be moments like that at school that you don't see?

Two points here: One, children may learn different things in different settings, and the "eureka" moments we see from one-to-one teaching are a qualitatively different kind of learning than the accretion and consolidation of increasing competencies that can come from being part of a group and a routine. Think of one-to-one learning as steps, one higher than the next, and group learning as more of a smooth curve. Two, you need to understand how to support your child through both these types of learning experiences—if they are right for his learning differences and stage of development.

How can you help your child's teachers and therapists do the best job they can? How can you best support teachers both psychologically and substantively? You already know that research supports the idea that interventions involving parents are among the most successful ones. In my experience, this means that parents need to understand their children's therapies well enough to be able to talk about the concepts involved and to understand how what they do at home with their child can support and hopefully even enhance the work of professionals.

Supporting Home Programs

Parents with home programs open their homes to tutors and their various supervisors. For certain this means having a countertop coffee carafe and snacks for team meetings, but what else? How are you a part of this team? Do you provide the examples of when Jerome wouldn't pull up his pants—even though you know it's been "mastered"—and begged for help? That's okay. But more should be expected from you.

As Jerome's mom, you may be the only one in a position to realize that he won't pull up pants with a drawstring or when he also has his shoes on. Any ideas to share with the group on how to get him through that? Stronger visual supports for what he must do when it's time for "pants up"? A written sign that says "Pants Up!"? A reward for going potty that doesn't come till pants are up? You can think of this stuff as well as they can! Don't feel that some twenty-two-year-olds who've been at this a couple of years have all the answers. Sure, they can package it into a "pants up program." But don't forget that if Jerome weren't autistic, you'd still need to teach him to pull his pants up, and you wouldn't have four concerned twenty-two-year-olds and their thirty-something supervisor to help you.

In addition to strategic support (such as contributing knowledge of what pants your child prefers), you can provide material support. This means doing some one-to-one work yourself—for your own buy-in. You need to convince yourself of your self-efficacy with your child's learning as well as show your child you can be a shaper of her behavior. This latter point is particularly important. As a parent of a child who has been diagnosed with an autism spectrum disorder, you have had more than your share of experiences where your child did not respond to your natural parenting efforts as robustly as other children. It's hard to imagine someone who does not take this personally on some conscious or unconscious level—and have to overcome some sense of being less than a good-enough parent.

Supporting Classroom Teachers

Most parents of typically developing preschoolers volunteer at school. This has several benefits: On one hand, it enriches the adult-to-child ratio, giving every pupil opportunities for more individual attention and freeing the teacher to teach more and manage less. On the other hand, the parent gets to see what other children the same age are like and learn strategies for encouraging development and managing behavior as done by a pro. In elementary school, especially the early elementary grades, parents often do essentially the same thing for the same reasons. So why so much less in special education? These kids need more help, not less!

We've just finished enumerating ways that parents who put in time in their child's ABA/DTT program are better positioned to find ways to practice and extend emerging skills through daily opportunities. The same thing can be true of helping at school. Even if you just hang out and guide a couple of kids to set the table for snack, cut out construction-paper Easter bunnies for art, or are playground or lunch monitor once a week, you can learn a lot. You might even learn to help pupils "Check Your Schedule!" What's more, you'll see how your child functions as part of a group. You may learn a thing or two about how a small physical prompt or redirect to a visual support can help things click and get your child to stay with everyone else. Another advantage is that you'll see your child's teacher in action. She'll get comfortable having you around. She will have to respect your time in class; you'll inevitably learn to respect her when you see how much there is to do. When you have your next IEP meeting, you won't be strangers.

When Does Mom or Dad Get an Apple?

Mom or Dad gets two apples, actually: The all-important benefit of knowing how to work effectively with your child yourself is that it positions you perfectly to understand what to teach your child next. Parents who know their child's interests, vocabulary, and grammar intimately are the ones who can find the natural opportunities to reinforce lessons being learned in more formal instruction.

Second, if you can truly be part of your child's team—either in a home program or at school—you have a secure, legitimate basis for trust, respect, and dialogue with your professional service providers. It's one thing to have a "legal" right to this. It's another to earn respect by taking responsibility for your child yourself and giving back to the system that helps your child.

Communicating Concern
If You Think Treatment Isn't Working

Not every treatment you select will work. Your child may change and have new or different treatment needs. The helping professionals may change, other children in your child's class may change, and the composition of services will certainly change with each year's new IEP. When you can see that things are not working well, you'll need to develop ideas about why that is and communicate your observations to teachers, therapists, or school administrators who are involved. Don't start off by using certified mail—or use Express Mail or FedEx either. Call the person closest to the issue and ask if you can get together and talk at a mutually convenient time. Start with a small meeting and a level playing field, preferably just two people, to make your concern seem as small and readily solvable as possible.

If your problem is with an aide or tutor, this is someone who should basically be doing what his supervisor tells him, so talk to his supervisor first. Don't call in the aide or tutor at this point; it will only make him worried and anxious that he isn't carrying out his job responsibilities satisfactorily. From the point of view of retaining him to continue to work (well) with your child, it's much better to leave him out of the loop until a positive plan for a new direction to be tried is devised.

If your problem is with the content of your child's program or the methods being used, talk to the teacher or program manager—in other words, the person responsible for the curriculum. Start any meeting with some comments about what you feel is going well. Be prepared to offer solutions, not just criticisms. Then get to your concerns about what's not going so well. Try to think of solutions that don't simply discard what you have for something else but to make what you have into what you think your child needs.

Try to back up your statements with concrete support. For example, saying "I don't think Sarah likes coming to school anymore" begs the question "What makes you think so?" If Sarah is crying more in the afternoons, maybe something that's going on in the afternoon should be considered as an alternative explanation. Discuss all alternative explanations for a problem. See if you can anticipate explanations you might get for your concerns and consider the possible validity of these.

If you suggest modifications that a therapist or teacher can't offer, or argues is not needed, you'll need to take the matter further. If you and the teacher or program manager can't figure out where to go with your discussion, agree on how to widen the circle of advisers for the issue. Maybe a teacher would want a second meeting involving the resource specialist. Maybe a speech and language pathologist would want to do new language testing to gauge exactly where your child is if you think he understands more and she thinks he understands less. A home ABA/DTT program manager might bring in her program director if you feel your son's drills are boring him and she feels he just hasn't mastered them.

If you find that a professional acts defensively, try not to escalate—though it can be hard. You could try reminding her that this is about understanding how Matthew learns and what else might be tried. See if you can identify with part of her position. Let her tell you the things she has considered and tried to address your issue.

If a second meeting is needed, try to manage the escalation. If there will be two people from the school or service agency, take your spouse or other support person with you. Meetings with casts of thousands accomplish little anyway, and most people don't really need to be there and will end up saying little or nothing.

Transition Planning

Sometimes things go wrong because of a new program or service provider that hasn't worked out as planned. If the old thing was still working, maybe you can just go back to it. Moving a child along due to chronological age is pretty silly when you're teaching to a developmental age that is rather different. (I'm an "If it ain't broke, don't fix it" kind of gal.) If there is no going back, perhaps the former, successful provider can consult with the new one.

In any case, transition planning should be carried out to anticipate difficulties that can result from introduction of new services. It's true that children with autism can on average have more difficulties with even trivial changes than typically developing children. However, special education case law has made a massive mess of this, enshrining transition planning in a way that goes way beyond what current research can support.

All kids like to know what to expect. All kids want to know what's happening and why—whether or not they have any choice in the matter. These topics are the fodder of many an argument and tantrum between parents and toddlers, preschoolers, and school-age children. Autistic children are no different. It's only that they get more upset at changes because they generally cannot use language to understand what's happening. Even if they can use language, logic and analogous thinking tend to be more than a little bit weak. This is compounded by the autistic desire to please oneself over others. So, okay, yes, transitions can be a problem for children with autism spectrum disorders.

However, I have been a consultant on numerous IEPs and even given testimony in due process hearings where transition plans of six months or more are proposed to move a child from, say, a home program to a school program. This sort of thing, of course, is just a thin guise for keeping a child in a home program and out of school—even when unique benefits of the more restrictive home program can no longer be demonstrated (and there just might be a good thing or two to adapting to life outside one's den/bedroom/classroom).

What's a good transition then? A child starting a new class might initially go there from another one with a familiar aide for one or two familiar activities a week. After a month, maybe a few mornings a week can be spent in the new program with a familiar aide. Three is my magic number for how many times per week a child needs to attend a program that others attend full-time in order to begin to be part of the new group. The same is true with respect to transitioning from a home to a school program.

As soon as a child starts to transition, consider whether any individualized support staff should accompany your child for the transition. This means that a one-to-one tutor from a home program, shadowing a child in preschool, might be gradually replaced by someone from the preschool to assist the child in becoming a more full member of his new group. Some children who rely on equal or almost equal amounts of home and school programming might benefit from one aide who is the same in both settings to provide continuity and consistency of programming. Otherwise, periodic visits of staff from one site to the other or joint team meetings can help meet this need for continuity.

One of the biggest problems in transitioning comes about when staff in each of two settings where a child receives services do things differently. That's okay. Different can be okay. In fact, it's really important to give a child with autism opportunities to use emerging skills in multiple settings. A behaviorist would call this "generalizing." You might also want to call it "meaningful acquisition." As long as each setting is developmentally and methodologically suited to the child's learning needs, it should be safe sailing.

Will My Child Regress? What's *Recoupment*?

An issue related to transitions and transition planning is that of regression and recoupment. The term *regression* used here refers to the concern that a child with an autism spectrum disorder may be more liable to lose skills when there is either a loss of continuity in instruction or a hiatus in instruction. The term *recoupment*, introduced in Chapter 9, refers to how long it takes to recover skills presumably lost during a hiatus. Some recoupment is expected for all kids: Typical kindergarteners spend the year learning the alphabet, upper and lower case, the sounds the letters make, blends, vowel sounds, and so on. Then, during the first month of first grade (after a typical ten-week hiatus for summer break), they spend the first month of first grade "learning" these exact same things—a one-month recoupment period when not much new is being introduced and they are just consolidating what they learned last year.

Regression is a pretty scary thing for parents of any developmentally delayed child to contemplate, and particularly traumatizing for the 15–30% of parents of children with autism who see their children lose words, social skills, and play interests they once clearly had. This has made the specter of regression due to summer breaks an area of real concern in both transition planning and hiatuses of service for children with autism. Most children with autism learn slower, forget faster, and take longer to consolidate and retain new information to begin with. A ten-week summer vacation would likely necessitate a month more of recoupment for most newly acquired skills than it does with typically developing children the same age. Even the six weeks between the end of the Extended School Year (ESY) and the beginning of the next might be a problem. However, this is all really "broad brushstrokes" talk because there is no body of research that completely applies here.

Is four days off from services for Thanksgiving (twice as much as a weekend!) too much? What about a week for Easter? Is two weeks off for Christmas and New Year's okay? How about six weeks between the end of the ESY and the beginning of the next? Answer? It depends on the child. It depends on how newly established the skills that won't get practice are. As a rule of thumb, the newer the skills, the less of a break from instruction there should be: A newly diagnosed child starting services of any type for the first time in early June is not likely to be well served by six weeks off after his first six weeks on. A nonverbal, moderately retarded eight-year-old who needs a highly routinized and visually structured setting might have problems with even two weeks off. These are examples of the kinds of children for whom breaks should be minimized per the IEP.

What should you be doing to ameliorate the effect of breaks you may feel are too long? The best answer from the point of view of the child's welfare is to think of ways you can step up and provide continuity in structure at home (which largely should be in place anyway), short of running a mini-classroom from your child's bedroom. Regular school holidays afford families the opportunity for special activities, and to the extent reasonable, your family should reach for this too. Get a pass to Disneyland that lets kids with disabilities go to the front of the line. Take a babysitter along when you go to a restaurant or movie so the sitter and your child can step out or leave if your child gets "toasted." Of course, school also serves a respite function when it comes to helping a more high-needs child. Additional respite care, visual supports that can be added at home, a daily routine that parents and teachers can realistically work out together, special activities with high interest (like playground time, more than usual TV/video time) can all fill in.

When it comes to school-age children particularly, we certainly have no evidence that neurons only partly activated for a couple weeks of a break in services will shrivel from their synapses. It is, in fact, rather unlikely in an eight-year-old. The bigger concern during breaks is that your child will capitalize on a change in supports to try to do things the "easy" way—screaming, running, not complying—rather than finding words and following with practiced expectations. If these things are successful during a break, precious teaching time will be lost when services resume and your child has to readjust to firmer demands. Each child's case is individual and depends on the child's current rate on the learning curve, her age, supports available through her home, and related factors. One hopes that children with autism can have vacations too—have a chance to do some things with their families (even if not all things can be tolerated) and a chance for some time off to learn in the informal way that children can learn when exposed to novel experiences.

Summing Up Your Rights and Responsibilities

In this chapter, we discussed how you can develop productive relationships with the people who help you help your child. These relationships start when you look for services and open your first dialogues with people who may be the ones to teach or give therapy to your child. These relationships need to be founded in mutual trust, two-way communication, and a sense on your part that what you put into the system will filter through to the quality of care your child may be expected to receive. A child with an IEP has many enshrined rights. The child who is likely to be well served is the one whose parents, as well as professionals, are each and all altruistic citizens of his community.

You've got some work ahead. Done well, there is no doubt that it can offer a better future ahead for your child. The best way out is up. After reading all this, you're ready to launch. As Buzz Lightyear would say: "To infinity and beyond!"

Resources

Books for Parents

Other Books for Parents and Professionals by Bryna Siegel

Siegel, B. (1996). *The world of the autistic child: Understanding and treating autistic spectrum disorders.* New York: Oxford University Press.

Siegel, B. (2003). *Helping children with autism learn: Treatment approaches for parents and professionals.* New York: Oxford University Press.

Siegel, B., & Silverstein, S. (1994). *What about me?: Growing up with a developmentally disabled sibling.* New York: Insight Books, Plenum Press. (Republished by Perseus Press).

Chapter 9 of this book, "Navigating the Legal Byways: Entitlements That Foster Learning," is available in a longer form with citations to relevant case law, and can be obtained from Kathryn E. Dobel at *spedlaw@comcast.net*. This version will be especially helpful to an advocate or special education attorney working with you in a matter that may be subject to administrative hearing under the IDEA.

On Understanding Autism Spectrum Disorders

Koegel, L. K., & LaZebnik, C. (2005). *Overcoming autism: Finding the answers, strategies, and hope that can transform a child's life.* New York: Penguin Books.

Ozonoff, S., Dawson, G., & McPartland, J. (2002). *A parent's guide to Asperger syndrome and high-functioning autism: How to meet the challenges and help your child thrive.* New York: Guilford Press.

Schreibman, L. (2005). *The science and fiction of autism.* Boston: Harvard University Press.

Szatmari, P. (2004). *A mind apart: Understanding children with autism and Asperger syndrome.* New York: Guilford Press.

On Families

Amenta, C. A., III. (1992). *Russell is extra special: A book about autism for children.* New York: Brunner/Mazel.
Grandin, T. (1995). *Thinking in pictures: And other reports from my life with autism.* New York: Doubleday.
Harris, S. L., & Glasberg, B. A. (1994). *Siblings of children with autism: A guide for families.* New York: Woodbine House.
Maurice, C. (1994). *Let me hear your voice: A family's triumph over autism.* New York: Ballantine Books.
Park, C. C. (2001). *Exiting Nirvana: A daughter's life with autism.* New York: Little, Brown.

On Comprehensive Therapy Approaches

Greenspan, S. I., & Wieder, S., with Simons, R. (1998). *The child with special needs: Encouraging intellectual and emotional growth.* Reading, MA: Addison-Wesley Longman.
Gutstein, S. C., & Sheely, R. K. (2002). *Relationship development intervention with young children: Social and emotional development activities for Asperger syndrome, autism, PDD and NLD.* New York: Jessica Kingsley.
Harris, S., & Handleman, J. (1994). *Preschool education programs for children with autism.* Austin, TX: PRO-ED.
Koegel, R. L., & Koegel, L. K. (Eds.). (1995). *Teaching children with autism: Strategies for initiating positive interactions and improving learning opportunities.* Baltimore: Brookes.
Lord, C. (Chair). (2001). *A report of the National Research Council: Educating children with autism.* Washington, DC: National Academy Press.
McClannahan, L. E., & Krantz, P. J. (1999). *Activity schedules for children with autism: Teaching independent behavior.* New York: Woodbine House.

On Behavioral Approaches

Baker, B. L., & Brightman, A. J. (1997). *Steps to independence: Teaching everyday skills to children with special needs* (3rd ed.). Baltimore: Brookes.
Harris, S. L., & Weiss, M. J. (1998). *Right from the start: Behavioral intervention for young children with autism.* Bethesda, MD: Woodbine House.
Leaf, R., & McEachin, J. (Eds.). (1999). *A work in progress: Behavior management strategies and a curriculum for intensive behavioral treatment of autism.* New York: DRL Books.
Lovaas, O. I. (1987). Behavioral treatment and normal educational and intellec-

tual functioning in young autistic children. *Journal of Consulting and Clinical Psychology, 55,* 3–9.

On Communication and Social Skills Approaches

Baker, J. E. (2003). *Social skills training for children and adolescents with Asperger syndrome and social–communication problems.* Shawnee, KS: Autism Asperger Publishing.

Koegel, R. L., & Koegel, L. K. (2006). *Pivotal response treatments for autism: Communication, social, and academic development.* Baltimore: Brookes.

Quill, K. A. (2000). *Do–watch–listen–say: Social and communication intervention for children with autism.* Baltimore: Brookes.

Resources in the United States

Autism Society of America (ASA)
7910 Woodmont Avenue, Suite 300
Bethesda, MD 20814-3067
Phone: 301-657-0881 or 800-3AUTISM
E-mail: *info@autism-society.org*
Website: *www.autism-society.org*

The ASA is the oldest and largest grassroots organization within the autism community. Today, more than 120,000 members and supporters are connected through a working network of nearly two hundred chapters nationwide.

The Centers for Disease Control and Prevention (CDC)
Autism Information Center
Website: *www.cdc.gov/ncbddd/autism/*

National Institute of Mental Health (NIMH)
Public Information and Communications Branch
6001 Executive Boulevard, Room 8184, MSC 9663
Bethesda, MD 20892-9663
Phone: 301-443-4513 or 866-615-6464
E-mail: *nimhinfo@nih.gov*
Website: *www.nimh.nih.gov/healthinformation/autismmenu.cfm*

The NIMH is one of twenty-seven components of the National Institutes of Health (NIH), the federal government's principal biomedical and behavioral research agency. NIH is part of the U.S. Department of Health and Human Services. The NIMH mission is to reduce the burden of mental illness and behavioral disorders through research on mind, brain, and behavior.

The Office of Special Education and Rehabilitative Services (OSERS)
U.S. Department of Education
400 Maryland Avenue, S.W.
Washington, DC 20202-7100
Phone: 202-245-7468
Website: *www.ed.gov/about/offices/list/osers/index.html*

Autism Resources
Website: *www.autism-resources.com*

   Links to numerous areas of autism resources for parents and teachers.

First Signs
P.O. Box 358
Merrimac, MA 01860
Phone: 978-346-4380
E-mail: *info@firstsigns.org*
Website: *www.firstsigns.org*

   Information on getting early screening and diagnosis for autism spectrum disorders.

Wrightslaw—Special Education
E-mail: *webmaster@wrightslaw.com*
Website: *www.wrightslaw.com/info/autism.index.htm*

   This Web page provides parents, advocates, educators, and attorneys with accurate, up-to-date information about special education law and advocacy so they can be effective catalysts.

Special Needs Project
342 State Street, Suite H
Santa Barbara, CA 93101
Phone: 800-333-6867
Website: *www.specialneedsproject.com*

   Excellent online bookstore for evidence-based books on understanding and treating autism.

International Resources

National Autistic Society, UK (NAS)
393 City Road
London EC1V 1NG United Kingdom
Phone: +44 (0)20 7833 2299
E-mail: *nas@nas.org.uk*
Website: *www.nas.org.uk*

Autism Spectrum Australia (ASPECT)
41 Cook Street
Forestville, NSW 2087
Australia
Phone: (02) 8977 8300
E-mail: *infoline@aspect.org.au*
Website: *www.aspect.org.au*

Autism Today
2016 Sherwood Drive, Suite 3
Sherwood Park, AB
T8A 3X3 Canada
Phone: 780-482-1555
E-mail: *info@autismtoday.com*
Website: *canadianautism.com*

Autism-Europe
Rue Montoyer 39
1000 Brussels, Belgium
Phone: +32(0)2 675 7505
E-mail: *secretariat@autismeurope.org*
Website: *www.autismeurope.org*

Autism-Europe plays a key role in raising public awareness and in influ-
encing the European decision makers on all issues relating to autism, including
the promotion of the rights of people with autism and other disabilities involving complex dependency needs.

Index

About the Author

Bryna Siegel, PhD, is Director of the Autism Clinic and Co-Director of the Autism and Neurodevelopment Research Center at the University of California, San Francisco. She has worked with children with autism and their families for 25 years, and has developed diagnostic tools and guidelines used by professionals nationwide. Dr. Siegel is an active lecturer and consultant whose previous books include the bestselling *World of the Autistic Child.*